Advance Praise for *Whole P*

"In this landmark book, Deborah Kesten and Larry Scherwitz have conducted, and are reporting revolutionary research proving for the first time, that replacing today's "new normal" overeating styles with their evidence-based Whole Person Integrative Eating program is a safe, scientifically sound step toward overcoming overeating and a lifetime struggle with weight. If people follow the revolutionary program outlined in this game-changing, insightful book, it may be the most helpful step they can take toward losing weight and keeping it off."

—Kenneth R. Pelletier, Ph.D., M.D.,
Clinical Professor of Medicine,
University of California School of Medicine, San Francisco;
author of *Change Your Genes, Change Your Life*

"*Whole Person Integrative Eating* is a masterful, holistic, integrative, and scientifically sound roadmap for overcoming overeating, overweight, and obesity. Deborah Kesten and Larry Scherwitz have written a breakthrough, evidence-based book that provides a clear guide for losing weight and keeping it off. Their practical science-backed advice will help the millions who struggle with weight issues. It ought to be mandatory reading in educational institutions. This is a must read."

—Marilyn Schlitz, Ph.D.,
Dean, Institute of Transpersonal Psychology at Sofia University;
President Emeritus and Senior Fellow at Institute of Noetic Sciences

"*Whole Person Integrative Eating* is not only a fascinating guide to choosing foods for health. It is a step-by-step plan to revolutionize your health."

—Neal D. Barnard, M.D., F.A.C.C., President,
Physicians Committee for
Responsible Medicine, Washington, D.C.

"As an endocrinologist and nutrition expert, I have reviewed numerous scientific and consumer publications regarding diet and nutrition. I have had major concerns that little attention has been paid to the emotional and lifestyle factors that influence the way we eat as well as what we eat. *Whole Person Integrative Eating* is a brilliant discourse on the root causes of overeating and ensuing weight gain that fills this gap. Authors Deborah Kesten and Larry

Scherwitz provide both scientific and realistic analyses of these issues, while offering practical, substantive, scientifically sound therapeutic suggestions. This excellent and unique book should be read widely by both health professionals and consumers."

—Leonard A. Wisneski, M.D., F.A.C.P.,
fellow, American College of Nutrition;
chair, Integrative Health Policy Consortium;
faculty, Georgetown University, George Washington University,
University of Colorado

"With *Whole Person Integrative Eating*, authors Deborah Kesten and Larry Scherwitz deliver a profoundly empowering program for losing weight and keeping it off. This evidence-based masterpiece not only educates but gives you an easy, precise strategy to experience sustainable freedom from the ravages of obesity. You will discover 1) insights and tools to diagnose why you overeat; 2) the treatment (cure) to your style(s) of overeating; 3) and deeper awareness and connection to the meaning of food and your own humanity. As an Internal Medicine physician with over two decades of experience in treating obesity, I am recommending this work to my patients without reservation."

—David Reed Miloy, M.D., M.S.,
founder, Optimum Health: Partners in Wellness;
life and wellness coach

"The program in *Whole Person Integrative Eating* is unique in that it brings consciousness to the experience of food and eating like no other approach. I know the Whole Person Integrative Eating (WPIE) program is effective, because I have applied it to patients with type 2 diabetes. My research revealed that the *how* components of WPIE (such as positive emotions, mindfulness, gratitude, etc.) were even more powerful determinants of lowering blood sugar levels than *what* participants ate. *Whole Person Integrative Eating* is a paradigm-changing program that takes the concept of nutritional health to a new level. With a deeper sense of personal nourishment, I believe it could help many overcome overeating, obesity, and other diet-related conditions."

—Ryan Bradley, N.D., M.P.H.,
Director of Research & Professor of Nutrition,
National University of Natural Medicine;
Professor of Preventive Medicine, University of California at San Diego

"This book will change your life. It is a personal guide to food wisdom that explains *what* to eat, *how* to eat, and *why* based on modern nutritional science and ancient food traditions that served us well for millennia. The authors unpack overeating and becoming overweight with remarkable clarity, sensitivity, and intelligence. In short, it is the most potent prescription available for healthful eating as a lifestyle choice."

—Peter Boland, Ph.D., President, Boland Healthcare;
visiting scholar, University of California at Berkeley

"*Whole Person Integrative Eating* is about much more than food, eating, and weight. I experienced the power of Whole Person Integrative Eating (WPIE) in my medical practice when I conducted research on WPIE with diabetic patients. When they applied the seven root causes of overeating that authors Deborah Kesten and Larry Scherwitz have identified, they were transformed. Confusing, conflicted relationships with food and eating become joyful again, and emotional and physical healing occurred. Overeating and obesity simply resolved as "side effects" of practicing Whole Person Integrative Eating, and turning to food to cope with unpleasant emotions was replaced with peace and self-compassion. This book shines a light on the path of self-discovery and healing."

—Erica Oberg, N.D., M.P.H.,
Naturopathic Doctor, Guarneri Integrative Health;
research scientist with more than 30 peer-reviewed published articles

"The flurry of recommendations for attaining and maintaining weight loss has for decades resembled an out-of-control food fight—a blizzard of competing, contrary advice that leaves people disappointed and demoralized. What a pleasure to see this science-based approach of Deborah Kesten and Larry Scherwitz. The program in *Whole Person Integrative Eating* honors *all* we are—not simply mindless eating machines, but many-faceted individuals whose physical, mental-emotional, social, cultural, historical, and spiritual characteristics play key roles in *every* aspect of food choice, consumption, metabolism, and health. Too complicated? Not really. Kesten and Scherwitz will lead you on a path that will leave you joyful, for two major reasons: this process feels good, and it works."

—Larry Dossey, M.D.,
author, *One Mind: How Our Individual Mind is Part of a Greater Consciousness
and Why It Matters*

"Because most chronic conditions are rooted in poor food choices, *Whole Person Integrative Eating* fills an important need: It provides a scientifically sound, unique, and enjoyable way to eat optimally, inspired by ancient food wisdom from great cultures and civilizations worldwide. Based on the authors' original research, *Whole Person Integrative Eating* presents a clear, step-by-step path to go from a way of eating that damages both our health and the health of our planet, to a relationship to food and eating that leads to overcoming overeating, overweight, and obesity. Highly recommended."

—Jean-Marc Fullsack,
Executive Chef/Instructor,
University of San Francisco School of Management;
Walter Reed Medal for Outstanding Performance,
Walter Reed Medical Center

"In *Whole Person Integrative Eating*, authors Deborah Kesten and Larry Scherwitz provide a research-based framework that is essential to understanding eating behaviors and the keys to optimal nourishment of the body and soul. This book broadens traditional views on weight management by taking a "whole person" approach. It is a must-read for those interested in how food and eating help to achieve and maintain well-being."

—Terri Merritt-Worden, M.S.,
Vice President, Operations - Blue Zones Project® by Sharecare

"Finally, a book that pops the major myth of weight loss. With their 7 styles of eating, Kesten and Scherwitz show that HOW you eat is just as important as WHAT you eat. Here are clear, step-by-step instructions on that HOW. It's all about the mindset and reading this book will change yours."

—Wayne B. Jonas, M.D.,
Executive Director, Samueli Integrative Health Programs;
author, *How Healing Works*

"*Whole Person Integrative Eating* serves as both a detailed guide to conscious eating and a complete support system for accomplishing this often-daunting task. What distinguishes this work from others I have seen and reviewed is that it addresses the needs of virtually all looking for guidance and guarantee of success for overcoming overeating and weight loss. As a naturopathic physician who started his career as a staff physician for Robert Atkins, confronting a myriad of dietary difficulties and well-intentioned but myopic guidelines from multiple sources, this work by Kesten and Scherwitz stands alone as a complete toolbox and resource grounded in both scientific rigor and pragmatic validity. I am delighted by their contribution and honored to add my hearty endorsement."

—Andrew L. Rubman, N.D.,
founder, Southbury Clinic for Traditional Medicines;
fellow, International Association for Medical Preventics

"By integrating emotions, relationships, and "spiritual ingredients" into the experience of food and eating, *Whole Person Integrative Eating* offers an alternative to the focus on just "what to eat" for weight loss, health, and healing. Supported by a multitude of studies and the authors' own original research, *Whole Person Integrative Eating* addresses the underlying biological, psychological, spiritual, and social causes of overeating, overweight, and obesity. Everyone can benefit from this "whole person" approach to managing and reversing food-related chronic conditions."

—David Riley M.D.,
Editor, *The Permanente Journal*;
founder, Scientific Writing in Health and Medicine (SWIHM)

ALSO BY DEBORAH KESTEN

Make Weight Loss Last
The Healing Secrets of Food
Feeding the Body, Nourishing the Soul

For more information about Whole Person Integrative Eating,
please go to www.IntegrativeEating.com
and www.MakeWeightLossLast.com.

Whole Person Integrative Eating

WHOLE PERSON
INTEGRATIVE EATING

A Breakthrough *Dietary Lifestyle* to
TREAT THE ROOT CAUSES
of Overeating, Overweight, and Obesity

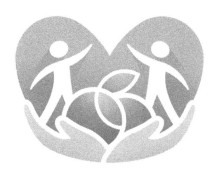

DEBORAH KESTEN, M.P.H.
LARRY SCHERWITZ, Ph.D.

Foreword by Dean Ornish, M.D.

White River Press
Amherst, Massachusetts

First published by
White River Press, PO Box 3561
Amherst, Massachusetts 01004
Whiteriverpress.com

ISBN: 978-1-887043-54-0 paperback | 978-1-887043-55-7 ebook

Cover design by María Clara León.
Book design by GPK industria gráfica Cuenca - Ecuador

Recipes reprinted with permission of the publisher from *The Pueblo Food Experience Cookbook: Whole Food of Our Ancestors* edited by Roxanne Swentzell and Patricia M. Perea (Museum of New Mexico Press, 2016).

This book is not meant as a substitute for medical advice and treatment from a physician or trained health professional. If you know or suspect you have a health problem, it is recommended that you seek your physician's advice before embarking on any program or treatment. The publisher and authors disclaim liability for any medical outcomes that may occur as a result of applying the methods suggested in this book.

Library of Congress Cataloging-in-Publication Data

Names: Kesten, Deborah, 1948- author. | Scherwitz, Larry, 1946- author.
Title: Whole person integrative eating : a breakthrough dietary lifestyle to
   treat the root causes of overeating, overweight, and obesity / Deborah
   Kesten, M.P.H. and Larry Scherwitz, Ph.D. ; foreword by Dean Ornish, M.D.
Description: Amherst, Massachusetts : White River Press, 2019. | Includes
   bibliographical references and index. |
Identifiers: LCCN 2019019408 (print) | LCCN 2019021859 (ebook) | ISBN
   9781887043557 (ebook) | ISBN 9781887043540 (pbk. : alk. paper)
Subjects: LCSH: Eating disorders--Popular works. | Eating
   disorders--Alternative treatment. | Eating disorders--Diet therapy. |
   Self-care, Health.
Classification: LCC RC552.E18 (ebook) | LCC RC552.E18 K48 2019 (print) | DDC
   616.85/26--dc23
LC record available at https://lccn.loc.gov/2019019408

Dedicated to Spirituality & Health *magazine,*
its first editor in chief Robert Owens Scott, and its readers.
Thank you for participating in national research on
Whole Person Integrative Eating.

CONTENTS

FOREWORD

For decades, modern nutritional sciences have been providing guidelines for what to eat and what not to eat for weight loss, health, and healing. Yet the advice about optimal eating often changes and can be confusing. Today, most of us know more about what doesn't work for the long term, like dieting, counting calories, and magical quick-fix solutions that promise rapid success.

Whole Person Integrative Eating offers an evidence-based alternative to the conventional wisdom about attaining and maintaining weight loss. Authors Deborah Kesten and Larry Scherwitz's Whole Person Integrative Eating (WPIE) dietary lifestyle—presented in this book—is a comprehensive, integrative, whole person program for enjoying food, weight loss, health, and healing, and addressing the underlying causes of overeating, overweight, and obesity. At the same time, this book brings to the table and to our daily lives ancient cultural wisdom that integrates both internal and external aspects of the eating experience so that body, mind, and soul are nourished each time we eat.

This program emerged when Kesten studied cross-cultural food- and nutrition-related guidelines, beliefs, and rituals by reviewing ancient food wisdom that had served humankind for millennia prior to the evolution of nutritional science in the twentieth century. By tracing the role of food through the wisdom traditions and by validating ancient food wisdom with modern nutritional science, Kesten and Scherwitz reveal that there is more to food than its ability to sustain us physically: it also nourishes us emotionally, spiritually, and socially. Our emotions, spiritual awareness, and social connections while eating play pivotal roles in how much we eat, how food is metabolized, and in turn how much we weigh.

More and more studies have documented that returning to what Kesten calls our "food roots"—going back to a diet of predominantly fresh, whole, plant-based foods—helps to prevent, manage, or even reverse a plethora of food-related chronic conditions, such as obesity, heart disease, diabetes, some cancers, depression, and more. Conversely, the more fast, animal-based, high-fat, high-sugar, and processed foods you consume, the more you're likely to overeat and be overweight or obese.

What's groundbreaking about Kesten and Scherwitz's research is twofold: They have created a scientifically sound, comprehensive, and integrative program for treating overeating, overweight, and obesity based on these principles.[1] And in addition to what we eat, they have identified seven statistically significant root reasons to explain why we overeat: what they call "new normal overeating styles" and eating behaviors that also have a profound influence on how much we eat and weigh.[2]

For instance, if you ever overeat to manage negative feelings, you're familiar with the Emotional Eating overeating style. But the other lesser known overeating styles—Food Fretting, Fast Foodism, Task Snacking, Sensory Disregard, Unappetizing Atmosphere, and Solo Dining—also have a profound influence on overeating and weight—plus on other diet-related chronic conditions.

For example, when diabetes researchers trained people with type 2 diabetes to replace their overeating styles with the Whole Person Integrative Eating dietary lifestyle Kesten and Scherwitz describe in this book, the researchers measured improvement in research participants' behaviors, including *how* they ate, which decreased and balanced blood-sugar levels even more than focusing only on *what* they ate.

The takeaway message in this well-researched and illuminating book is this: the antidote to overeating, overweight, and obesity and perhaps other diet-related chronic conditions may be to follow the ancient-food-wisdom-based guidelines that Kesten and Scherwitz describe in this book.

As Kesten writes, "The research on WPIE and the discovery of the overeating styles reveal that the reasons for overeating and weight gain are due to a newly identified complex of interconnected internal and external food and eating dynamics . . . . Identifying and modifying these dynamics and then nourishing the 'whole person' physically, emotionally, spiritually, and socially through WPIE may mean she or he does not need to compensate with overeating and satiety."[1]

In other words, by integrating the ancient physical, emotional, spiritual, and social dimensions of food, *Whole Person Integrative Eating* goes beyond the biochemical, what-to-eat ingredients in food. Rather, it offers a "whole person," evidence-based model and program that guide us to attaining and maintaining weight loss by nourishing ourselves with fresh, whole foods, but also with the nutrients missing from the food charts: positive emotions, mindfulness, appreciation, love, pleasant surroundings, and social connection. In this way, *Whole Person Integrative Eating* affirms the multidimensional healing power of food and leads us back to a deeper, healthier "whole person" relationship to food, eating, and weight loss.

Dean Ornish, M.D.
Founder & President, Preventive Medicine Research Institute
Clinical Professor of Medicine, University of California,
San Francisco

References:
1. Deborah Kesten and Larry Scherwitz, "Whole Person Integrative Eating: A Program for Treating Overeating, Overweight, and Obesity," *Integrative Medicine: A Clinician's Journal* 14, no. 5 (October/November 2015): 42–50.
2. Larry Scherwitz and Deborah Kesten, "Seven Eating Styles Linked to Overeating, Overweight, and Obesity," *Explore: The Journal of Science and Healing* 1, no. 5 (2005): 342–59.

ANCIENT FOOD WISDOM MEETS MODERN NUTRITIONAL SCIENCE

[Whole Person Integrative Eating] describes a new model of nutrition that merges ancient food wisdom with state-of-the-art science. [The] intriguing, well-researched message is that food influences . . . not only the physical dimensions of nutrition but also the emotional, spiritual, and social dimensions of what and how we eat.
—Dean Ornish, M.D., foreword to *The Healing Secrets of Food*[1]

The ancients knew something, which we seem to have forgotten.
—Albert Einstein

This is a book about overcoming overeating, overweight, and obesity by nourishing yourself physically, emotionally, spiritually, and socially each time you eat. The Whole Person Integrative Eating (WPIE) dietary lifestyle described in this book can help you transform your relationship with food and eating and in turn help you attain and maintain weight loss.

This program is based on overeating and obesity research that my co-author and husband, behavioral scientist Larry Scherwitz, Ph.D., and I have done during the past twenty-plus years. It is research that shows, for the first time, it may be possible for many people to overcome overeating and curtail weight gain simply by returning to their food roots: going back to a dietary lifestyle that nourished humankind physically, emotionally, spiritually, and socially for millennia.[2]

Using ancient food wisdom verified and supported by modern nutritional science, Larry and I discovered new normal food choices and eating behaviors linked to overeating, and we also discovered their antidote, the Whole Person Integrative Eating program we tell you about in this book. The more that participants in our study followed the ancient-food guidelines of Whole Person Integrative Eating, the more they enjoyed their food, the less they overate, and the more weight they lost—without dieting![2]

Unlike most traditional diets—meaning restrictive food regimens that end after a while—we are proposing a return to a way of eating, a "whole person" dietary lifestyle that is practiced for a lifetime.

As the incidence of overweight and obesity has been increasing during the past decades, so too have diseases linked to being obese, including heart disease, diabetes, hypertension, some cancers, metabolic syndrome, depression, and more. Yet if overeating, overweight, and obesity can be helped with a "whole person" dietary lifestyle, then it may also be preventable. Our research reveals that success depends not only on what you eat, but also on why, how, and with whom you eat on a daily basis. In other words, overeating and becoming overweight and obese may be both prevented and treated by a relationship to food and eating that nourishes physical, emotional, spiritual, and social well-being.[3] This book can help you tailor a personalized, Whole Person Integrative Eating program that is right for you.

This program does not require denial and deprivation, although it is likely an entirely different way of eating—a relationship to food that is unfamiliar to many. Our seventy-six-item questionnaire, "What's Your Overeating Style? Self-Assessment Quiz" (which is statistically validated, by the way, meaning it dependably predicts whether you overeat), introduces you to the multidimensional ingredients of Whole Person Integrative Eating.[1,4] After you take the quiz and determine your personal overeating styles, this book can help you make a decision about whether you have severe issues with overeating and would benefit from following all elements of the program or whether focusing on selected aspects would work better for you.

In other words, the program is not an all-or-nothing choice; rather, the degree to which it can help you enjoy food and take pleasure in the experience of eating, while decreasing food- and diet-related anxiety, stress, and the risk of overeating and weight gain, is your choice. At the same time, we're especially interested in telling you about the power of the Whole Person Integrative Eating dietary lifestyle to transform your relationship to food and eating in more meaningful, multidimensional ways.

The goal of the dietary lifestyle is not only to help you attain and maintain weight loss—although you likely will do so if you adopt it as a lifetime practice. On a deeper level, this book explores more than the physical aspect of what you eat and what you weigh; it also offers insights into the emotional, spiritual, and social dimensions of overeating and being overweight and obese. Our research revealed that being overweight and obese may be the visible manifestation of years of overeating, but for many, overeating often first begins in the mind (meaning, with the thoughts you think that lead to emotions you feel); soul (whether you live with a consciousness of heartfelt gratitude, mindfulness, and loving regard . . . or not); and whether you eat while surrounded by satisfying, supportive social connections . . . or not. In other words, overeating and ensuing weight gain are about more than calories in, calories out. They are influenced by the state of your psyche and spiritual and social dimensions.

Ultimately, the Whole Person Integrative Eating dietary lifestyle is about discovering what to eat to attain and maintain weight loss but also how to eat based on ancient food wisdom and insights from modern nutritional science: with positive feelings, mindfulness, gratitude, loving regard, and social connection. Twenty years ago, I may have said such changes in how you eat are difficult to measure scientifically, but this book is filled with studies that support each element of the Whole Person Integrative Eating program. Indeed, I'll tell you about some studies that have revealed these more invisible "ingredients" of the program may be more powerful determinants of your weight and well-being than what you eat.

Physically, the dietary lifestyle we tell you about in Whole Person Integrative Eating can help you choose optimal foods so you can begin to lose weight. Emotionally, it can help you to minimize and release negative emotions (such as anxiety and anger) when you eat and instead enjoy food filled with positive feelings (such as contentment and joy). Spiritually, it can help you to connect to your inner self by relating to food with mindfulness, gratitude, and love. And socially, it can help you to rediscover the healing power of dining with others as often as possible.

This program is a lifetime practice in how to take pleasure in food and eating. It is the opposite of dieting and deprivation in the traditional sense—how to relax and enjoy food, not how to stress over the "best" way to eat. How to stop judging yourself when you don't eat what you should. How to savor and be satisfied with the experience of eating, not fear food. How to eat with others in a pleasing atmosphere, not alone at your desk, while driving, or watching TV. In other words, how to nourish yourself physically, emotionally, spiritually, and socially each time you eat so that all of you, the whole person, can heal.

Ultimately, this is a book about creating a pleasurable, positive, balanced relationship to food and eating. Once that is done, losing weight and keeping it off is a secondary benefit, a side effect. We'll introduce you to the "new normals," the seven (statistically significant) overeating styles we've discovered, which have evolved during the last few decades, that are making us overweight,[2] and the antidote to the overeating styles—our Whole Person Integrative Eating dietary lifestyle.[3] Ultimately, what we're showing you is how to catch up with your culinary past so that you can claim your normal-weight heritage now. This book is divided into three sections:

Part One begins with an overview of our research about what this program can do for you. In these chapters, we describe the overeating styles and their link to weight, but also the biological, psychological, spiritual, and social elements of WPIE and weight. These aspects of WPIE have been written about piecemeal over the years, but for the most part they have been largely ignored in the weight-loss literature. Yet through our research and the studies of others, more and more I have come to understand that our emotions, connecting to the spiritual significance in food, and pleasant comradery while eating play key roles in weight-loss success and well-being. By telling you about our research, my intention is to up your understanding about what the WPIE dietary lifestyle can do for you when you "flavor" your daily meals with its "ingredients."

I'll also explain the seven overeating styles we've identified—what I call today's "new normals"—that contribute to overeating, overweight, and obesity. For example, I will explain why "Fast Foodism"— eating mostly fast and processed food—leads to weight gain, but also how and why "Food Fretting" (dieting and obsessing about the "best" way to eat), "Task Snacking" (eating while doing other activities), and other overeating styles may cause problems.

Perhaps most important, so you can identify your own personal root causes of overeating, we've created the "What's Your Overeating Style? Self-Assessment Quiz."[1,4] Recognizing and reflecting on the overeating styles will empower you to co-create your own personalized Whole Person Integrative Eating dietary lifestyle so you can live the balanced, healing relationship to food and eating you truly desire. Thus, when you identify which of the seven key styles of overeating you engage in, you'll have the tools and insights you need to address overeating, overweight, and obesity and to replace your overeating styles with a meaningful whole person relationship to food. In this way, identifying and examining your overeating styles may be the most important first step you can take to obtain and maintain weight loss.

But before you begin the program—which is a step-by-step guide to the Whole Person Integrative Eating dietary lifestyle—I'll help you enhance your success by introducing you to the "stages of change." This integrative, transtheoretical model of behavior change will give you the tools and insights you need to assess your readiness to take action and follow the WPIE program; to decide if you are ready to make the changes that are best for you personally and that can help you overcome overeating and increase your odds of weight loss.

Part Two gives you detailed descriptions of each of the seven elements of the Whole Person Integrative Eating dietary lifestyle, the antidotes to the overeating styles. Each chapter is replete with how-to, step-by-step guidelines for implementing each remedy. In these chapters, I'll describe and clarify the physical, emotional, spiritual, and social aspects of overeating and overweight, using ancient food wisdom and modern nutritional science studies. In other words, in this section, I'll present the whole person treatment for each overeating style and a detailed understanding of the research that supports each solution.

But before you begin the program, I'll help you enhance your success by demystifying what a Whole Person Integrative Eating "dietary lifestyle" actually is, and how it differs from the same ol', same ol' go-on-a-diet-then-gain-back-the-weight approach. Instead, Part Two will give you the tools and insights you need to follow the program by profoundly changing your relationship to food so that eating becomes one of life's greatest pleasures.

Part Three is replete with recipes that show you how to activate two key optimal what-to-eat concepts of the program: 1) eating fresh, whole foods 2) and "inverse eating," a centuries-old way of eating—validated by a plethora of today's scientific studies—that can help you stop the slide into overeating and obesity and its family of related conditions. To put the WPIE what-to-eat principles into action, I'll give you one week of menus chock-full of delicious international recipes—with both traditional and not so traditional versions.

As a nutrition and health researcher, I write this book filled with compassion for the millions who struggle with overweight and obesity and the distressing chronic conditions that often accompany them. My intention in writing this book is to share with you a scientifically sound, satisfying *dietary lifestyle* that can help you attain and maintain weight loss . . . for life. Yes, the elements of the Whole Person Integrative Eating program can empower you to make informed food and eating choices that can lead to weight loss, but my even bigger wish for you is that the foundational elements and philosophy of Whole Person Integrative Eating become a lifetime *practice*; a pleasurable journey you embark on each time you eat, revealing delight-filled culinary vistas that you visit daily.

The persistent story about those who succeed at weight loss focuses on eating less and moving more. With the integration of ancient food wisdom and modern nutritional science, *Whole Person Integrative Eating* adds additional dimensions to conventional wisdom by revealing that ingredients of weight-loss success may be more complex—and remarkable—than we've been led to believe.

In short, this book provides a comprehensive personal system—the Whole Person Integrative Eating dietary lifestyle—that helps to heal root causes of overeating, overweight, and obesity. As you familiarize yourself with the ancient food wisdom and practice the guidelines supported by modern nutritional science, see how you're feeling—physically, emotionally, spiritually, and socially. It is our hope that the program helps you to transform your relationship to food, eating, and weight and in the process find true nourishment . . . for life.

PART ONE

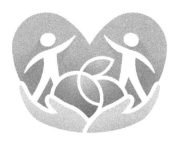

Whole Person Integrative Eating:
A Re-Visioning of Nutritional Health

CHAPTER 1

DISCOVERING WHOLE PERSON INTEGRATIVE EATING

[Whole Person Integrative Eating] provides a fresh perspective on our epidemic of overeating, overweight, and obesity. [It] identifies underlying causes of overeating and ensuing weight gain that, if replicated, could signal a paradigm shift in the field of nutrition.

—David Riley, M.D., "Integrative Nutrition: Food's Multidimensional Power to Heal"[1]

At the start of our coaching sessions, Alison was a single, five-foot-five, sixty-four-year-old Caucasian woman who weighed 265 pounds, her highest weight ever. A former businesswoman turned professional meditation practitioner, her weight gain, which had begun as a pre-teen, had continued to escalate in the following decades of her life.[2,3]

As we talked, I learned that Alison had called me after reading "The Enlightened Diet," an article I had written for *Spirituality & Health* magazine.[4] In the piece, I invited people to participate in an eighteen-lesson, six-week online course on Whole Person Integrative Eating (WPIE), a comprehensive program that addresses not only *what* to eat for physical health and healing but also *how* to eat for emotional, spiritual, and social nourishment—the four whole person facets of food that compose the WPIE dietary lifestyle we're telling you about in this book.

Alison was especially interested in the bio-psycho-spiritual-social approach of Whole Person Integrative Eating, because it fit her worldview and long-practiced contemplative meditation practices.

Weary from her lifetime struggle with obesity, she had tried many "diets du jour" over the decades—from high protein, low fat and low carb, to high fat, counting calories, eating "good" food and avoiding "bad" food, and doing a "detox" liquid-only regimen—the list goes on and on. And on. Each time she would lose some weight—sometimes a lot; then she would return to her preferred go-to foods and gain back the weight . . . and more. At the same time, her obesity-related ailments continued: high blood pressure, elevated cholesterol levels, pre-diabetes, and depression and anxiety. Even before she blurted, "I'm so frustrated!" I could hear the defeat and exasperation in her voice.

Alison had already figured out what would never, ever work for her: dieting and its twin, calorie counting. "Every time I eat those small portions of '*should*' food I don't enjoy, I feel angry and hopeless and so alone. When I'm dieting, I clear out all the foods I like to overeat so I'm not tempted—but every day I miss them; then, when I start to crave them, I give in. Meditation and spirituality have become a big part of my life now, so I resonate deeply with the idea of bringing more meaning to my meals, to relating to food in a different way so that food and eating are fulfilling—not something I fear, count, and obsess about. Does this make sense?"

Absolutely, I assured her. As a matter of fact, Alison was spot on with her realization that traditional dieting—which I define as a pre-scribed, regimented way of eating—isn't an effective solution for her to attain and maintain weight loss for the long term. This is because most people who lose weight tend to regain it, as Alison did. At the same time, a well-controlled study reveals that pounds lost appear about equal across the popular diet approaches, ranging from a low-fat, high-complex-carbohydrate diet to a high-protein, low-carbohydrate diet.[5,6]

When Alison contacted me, she already understood that such studies on dieting were verifying her personal experience: it does not seem to matter which diet overweight people follow; that over-eating, overweight, obesity, and other diet-related chronic conditions will not be solved with a singular focus on what and how much to eat. Might our evidence-based Whole Person Integrative Eating pro-gram—which addresses not only what to eat but also Alison's phys-ical, emotional, spiritual, and social well-being—bring to meals the meaning she sought and in turn bring sustainable weight loss and well-being?

The WPIE Intervention

Both Alison and I understood that changing her relationship to food, eating, and weight would not be easy. After all, it meant she would need to create (recreate?) a never-before-considered dietary lifestyle—a completely new relationship to food and eating that nourished her multidimensionally. "I'm ready to do this," Alison told me. "All that dieting and obsessing about food for decades hasn't worked; it's only made me miserable. I don't want to live like this anymore."

"I understand," I told her. "The eat-less, move-more prescription has helped many manage their weight, but I think that you personally will resonate strongly with an integrative way of eating that nourishes *all* of you each time you eat. I'm saying this because our WPIE program will give you the insights and skills you need to increase your odds of losing weight and keeping it off." I paused to make a key point: "And then there's this for you to mull over, Alison: Whole Person Integrative Eating is a lifetime practice—not a diet you go on, then off."

Alison considered what I was saying, then asked if I thought she would likely lose weight as a "natural side effect" of this new relationship to food and eating. "That's the intention," I responded. Still, given Alison's failed history of traditional yo-yo dieting—losing weight, then regaining even more—I realized how (understandably) apprehensive she was.

Over the next twelve months, I turned to the details of our original research to coach Alison in the Whole Person Integrative Eating dietary lifestyle.[3,7] We began with her filling out our "What's Your Overeating Style? Self-Assessment Quiz" to identify her unique food choices and eating behaviors that were leading her to overeat and to gain weight;[8] then, step-by-step, we replaced each of her overeating styles with the seven elements of the Whole Person Integrative Eating dietary lifestyle[3] I tell you about in Part Two of this book. Alison decided to begin her transformation by replacing the Unappetizing Atmosphere overeating style with eating in an Amiable Ambiance; see chapter 11 for more about this.

At the beginning of the year's coaching intervention, Alison weighed 235 pounds and wore a size 3X; one year later, she weighed approximately 165 pounds and wore a size 12. She has kept the weight off for five years.

Alison has attributed her weight loss to the "wholeness" of the Whole Person Integrative Eating dietary lifestyle she learned—and continues to practice. I believe she was successful because she was empowered by a scientifically sound self-care dietary lifestyle that nourished her physically, emotionally, spiritually, and socially: ergo, Whole Person Integrative Eating. By following her spot-on intuition—which for Alison meant infusing meaning into meals and replacing calorie counting with "whole person nourishment"—she achieved the naturally occurring weight loss she'd been seeking for years.

Here's the research story behind the Whole Person Integrative Eating model and program that led to Alison's weight-loss success. I'll give you step-by-step details of this ancient (and new) dietary lifestyle in Part Two, "The Whole Person Integrative Eating Dietary Lifestyle." First, here's a look at the current diet and obesity data, then the research story behind the Whole Person Integrative Eating dietary lifestyle as a path to overcoming overeating, overweight, and obesity.

Where We Are Now . . .

Even though nutritional science has made amazing discoveries about food, nutrition, health, and healing—especially during the last few decades—the prevalence of diet-related chronic conditions continues to surge. From obesity, diabetes, and cardiovascular disease to some cancers, ischemic stroke, metabolic syndrome, osteoporosis, and more, chronic conditions linked to diet have been skyrocketing for decades. Today, 133 million Americans (one in two Americans) suffer from chronic conditions, many of which are linked to food choices, and if trends continue, the number is projected to grow to about 157 million by 2020 and to 171 million by 2030.[9]

The prevalence of obesity especially is daunting, with 68 percent of adults in the United States either overweight or obese, as are one-third of children and adolescents.[10] Overweight and obesity significantly increase the risk of death from a range of related chronic conditions.[11] Indeed, for the first time in two centuries, due to the prevalence of chronic conditions, life expectancy in the United States is projected to decline.[12]

As most of you know, weight-loss programs and traditional dieting, which I'm defining as "a prescribed, regimented way of eating" that often includes curtailing calories, may have helped many lose weight, but they have not been an effective solution for resolving our obesity pandemic.

In my opinion, most traditional diets lead to weight loss because of the foods (actually, food *products*) they restrict, such as fried food, high-sugar and high-fat snacks, soft drinks, and so on. When most people stop the restrictive food regimen, they traditionally return to their go-to foods and way of eating. Because of this dynamic, the guesstimate of researchers is that between 80 to 95 percent of people who lose weight regain it. The elephant in the room is this: the real issue is what most of us typically eat every day. In other words, the foods we return to when we're not dieting is why we gain—and regain weight when we're not dieting.

The Genesis of Whole Person Integrative Eating

The idea to explore a multidimensional, ancient-food-wisdom approach to food and eating had its genesis in New Delhi, India, where my co-author and husband, behavioral scientist Larry Scherwitz, Ph.D., had been invited to present at the First International Conference on Lifestyle and Health. While there, I had the opportunity to interview clinical cardiologist Dr. K. L. Chopra—father and mentor of Deepak Chopra, M.D., who is an integrative-medicine and personal-transformation pioneer—about a magazine article I was intending to write on yoga and diet. When I asked Dr. Chopra about this, his response was immediate: "*Prana* is the vital life force of the universe, the cosmic force . . . and it goes into you, into me, with food. When you cook with love, you transfer the love into the food and it is metabolized . . . In former days (based on the Hindu scripture, the *Bhagavad Gita*), the tradition was for the mother to cook the food with love and then feed it to the children; only then would she eat."[13]

Food and love. The thought wouldn't let go. My thinking: if Hindus believe that loving awareness is somehow transmuted into food—and that we "ingest" this vital force when we eat—then possibly other spiritual traditions would have discovered this too. As a nutrition researcher, I was fascinated by the possibility that consciousness could alter the food we eat. And, I wondered, might it also influence metabolism of food and in turn health and healing? To find out, I began what I call my "nutrition journey around the world."

An Ancient Food Wisdom Odyssey: Moving Forward by Looking Back

For millennia prior to the birth of nutritional science in the twentieth century, humankind turned to the wisdom traditions—world religions, cultural traditions, and Eastern healing systems—for guidelines about what and how to eat. Given this, my quest led me to unearth and unravel cross-cultural food and nutrition guidelines, beliefs, and rituals from both the East and West. These include the following:

1. **Major world religions** (i.e., Judaism, Christianity, Islam, Hinduism, Buddhism)
2. **Cultural traditions** (i.e., yogic nutrition, African-American soul food, Native American beliefs, the Japanese Way of Tea, Chinese food folklore)
3. **Eastern healing systems** that include food and nutrition guidelines (i.e., traditional Chinese medicine, Ayurvedic medicine, Tibetan medicine)
4. **Nutritional science studies** (from research scientists worldwide)

Results from my research, which also includes interviews with more than fifty scientists, religionists, and spiritual experts, were published in my first book, *Feeding the Body, Nourishing the Soul*.[13]

An Old-New View: 6 Principles, 4 Facets of Food

When Larry and I stepped back to make sense of the enormous amount of ancient food wisdom we had amassed, we realized it encompasses six perennial principles that in turn comprise four facets *of food* (the focus of my second book, *The Healing Secrets of Food*).[14] In other words, ancient food wisdom provides guidelines for *1) biological* (what to eat for physical health), *2) psychological* (how food affects feelings), *3) spiritual* (the life-giving meaning in meals), *4) and social* (dining with others) nourishment: ergo, Whole Person Integrative Eating.

Here's how the six cohesive guidelines look from the perspective of the four facets:

Biological Nutrition

1. Eat fresh, whole foods in their natural state as often as possible.

Psychological Nutrition

2. Be aware of feelings and thoughts before, during, and after eating.

Spiritual Nutrition

3. Bring moment-to-moment nonjudgmental awareness to every aspect of the meal.
4. Appreciate food and its origins—from the heart.
5. Savor and "flavor" food with loving regard.

Social Nutrition

6. Unite with others through food.[3,14]

The six perennial principles and four facets of food tell us what religions, cultural traditions, and Eastern healing systems discovered instinctively and intuitively and what modern researchers are beginning to conjecture: that food empowers us to heal multidimensionally.

Ancient Food Wisdom Meets Modern Nutritional Science

Clearly, our research revealed that, for millennia, humankind and theologies turned to food to nourish physical, emotional, spiritual, and social well-being. The four facets of food reconnect us to this timeless food wisdom. Throughout this book, I'll be telling you about the four facets and perennial principles and the multitude of state-of-the-art studies that support each element and link them to health and healing. Here's a closer look at each facet and what it means to you.

Biological Nutrition. If you've ever chosen a particular food after calculating its calorie, carb, or fat-gram content—perhaps with the intention of maintaining or losing weight—or selected a particular food for its health-enhancing nutrients, such as antioxidants, you've experienced the biological or physical facet of food. Biological Nutrition explores the power of balanced nutrients (such as vitamins, minerals, antioxidants, phytochemicals, etc.) in fresh, whole food: the kind of food that our ancestors ate for millennia that has the power to heal versus today's new normal of fast, processed, denatured food, which can lead to weight gain and a multitude of ailments.

Psychological Nutrition. Do you ever wonder why you crave carrot cake instead of a carrot when you're, say, anxious? Psychological Nutrition is the facet of emotional well-being. It is an emerging field of mind-body nutrition research, which explores how food affects feelings via hormones (chemical messengers) that are released in the brain when we eat certain foods; and conversely, how thoughts and feelings often affect food choices.

Spiritual Nutrition. The spiritual facet of food explores three elements of awareness (*mindfulness*, *appreciation*, and *loving regard*) that we bring to the mystery of life inherent in food. The three elements of Spiritual Nutrition are the essence of the food-related wisdom espoused by world religions and cultural traditions for thousands of years. And eating with a spiritual consciousness influences digestion, health, and healing in a multitude of ways.

Social Nutrition. Think of a favorite food experience. Was it sharing food with some friends, family members, and coworkers, or were you dining at a table for one? This facet of social nourishment is about the health and healing benefits that food can bring when you're dining in a socially supportive environment.

In essence, the four facets of food Larry and I identified reveal that food has the power to nourish you not only physically but also emotionally, spiritually, and socially. In this way, the four facets provide a whole person relationship to food and eating. As you'll see throughout each chapter in Part Two about our Whole Person Integrative Eating program, each element holds the power to influence your health . . . and weight and well-being.

Definition: Whole Person Integrative Eating

With our discovery of the four facets of food, we believe a re-visioning of optimal dietary care is emerging. I coined the phrase "Whole Person Integrative Eating" to describe the four-facet way of eating, because the facets make connections between food and body, food and mind, food and soul, and food and social well-being.[4] Based on these findings, I define Whole Person Integrative Eating as a holistic, integrative approach to food, eating, health, and healing that addresses the power of food to heal multidimensionally.

At the same time, WPIE embraces evidence-based global nutrition guidelines and healing systems gleaned from many disciplines, with a special focus on nutritional anthropology, medical anthropology, and nutritional science. It is a model developed as an outcome of our research over the last two decades[1-4,6-8,13] and of our more recent study, which links *not* following each element of Whole Person Integrative Eating—our biological, psychological, spiritual, and social nutrition guidelines—to overeating, overweight, and obesity.[3,6]

At its core, we believe that WPIE reaffirms an optimal therapeutic relationship between food and eating, because it addresses whole person health and healing. Now Larry and I wanted to know if our Whole Person Integrative Eating model and program could help the millions who struggle with America's top health problems: overweight and obesity.

Does Whole Person Integrative Eating Influence Weight Loss?

The escalating prevalence of overweight and obesity in the U.S. is disheartening—for both the millions who struggle with weight and the health professionals who hope to help. Today, almost 32 percent of adults are overweight and nearly 40 percent are obese;[15] 15 percent of U.S. children are overweight and almost 17 percent are obese.[16] Such stats are of deep concern because being overweight escalates the risk for a range of other diet- and obesity-related chronic conditions—from diabetes and heart disease to metabolic syndrome, certain cancers, hypertension, and more.

To find out if there was a link between the perennial food wisdom Larry and I identified and its influence on weight, I partnered with *Spirituality & Health* magazine. In its cover story on the four facets of food and the six guidelines we identified, readers were invited to take my six-week, eighteen-lesson e-course on Whole Person Integrative Eating on the magazine's website.[17] Participants first completed our "What's Your Overeating Style? Self-Assessment Quiz?"[8,14]—and entered their height and weight. (You too can take the quiz in chapter 3.)

Of the 5,256 participants, throughout and after the e-course, those who increasingly ate according to the six perennial ancient-food themes were the ones who lost the most weight.

The New Normals: Meet the Overeating Styles

While the implications from our research are enormous in relation to the question of whether returning to our food roots and eating according to guidelines from ancient food wisdom could lead to weight loss, with another turn of our statistical kaleidoscope, we realized that the food choices and eating behaviors inherent in our seventy-six-item questionnaire could be clustered into seven styles of eating that *strongly* predict overeating and weight gain (see the appendix for more about this.) We call these "overeating styles," and we tell you about them in the next chapter, "Meet the Overeating Styles 'Family': 7 Root Causes of Overeating." They are:[7]

1. **Emotional Eating** (turning to food to self-medicate negative emotions)
2. **Fast Foodism** (consuming mostly denatured, processed food products)
3. **Food Fretting** (dieting and obsessing about the "best" way to eat)
4. **Task Snacking** (eating while doing other activities)
5. **Sensory Disregard** (eating without attention to flavors, aromas, presentation, etc.)
6. **Unappetizing Atmosphere** (eating in unpleasant *psychological* and *aesthetic* environments)
7. **Solo Dining** (eating alone more often than not)

If you take a close look at the seven overeating styles, it's clear they are all the new normal ways of eating for most Americans. After all, isn't eating mostly fast food—alone, often in unpleasant psychological or aesthetic surroundings, while experiencing negative emotions, multitasking and not focusing on food, or appreciating or "savoring flavors"—typical for most of us?

Our national study on the overeating styles, in which 5,256 individuals participated, revealed that these new normals matter a lot to your weight, because *all seven overeating styles are significantly and independently related to overeating frequency, and five of the seven are significantly related to being overweight or obese.*[7] In other words, the overeating styles identify and address *root reasons* many of us overeat and gain weight. Such findings suggest that *overeating is not merely an isolated behavior.* Rather, it is part of a complex web of related food choices, feelings, sensory experiences, and social behaviors that reflect the original meaning of the word *diet* as a way of life.

Viewed another way, all seven overeating styles strongly diverge from the perennial principles we've identified that served as eating guidelines in the past. These guidelines are the essence of the Whole Person Integrative Eating program we tell you about in Part Two of this book. Here's an essential key concept to keep in mind: The WPIE program isn't a black-or-white, all-or-nothing dietary lifestyle. Rather, all elements—from the new-normal overeating styles to the seven optimal-eating components of WPIE—occur on a continuum. The seven overeating styles and their opposite, the WPIE program, are two sides of the same coin.

Psychologist and obesity expert Kelly D. Brownell of the Rudd Center for Food Policy & Obesity at Yale University might explain our findings as "modern food conditions and their mismatch with evolution,"[18] because the essence of our findings is that there is a huge disparity between *what* (food choices) and *how* (eating behaviors) we eat today and what human beings ate and how they evolved for millennia.

In other words, as a society, we have systematically moved away from the time-tested, ancient, integrative modes of eating and living that kept us slimmer for centuries. The way we ate and lived for thousands of years seems to have kept us slender. The new normals—not only *what* we eat, but also the web of eating behaviors that identify *how* we have been eating and living for the past few decades—have not. (See chapter 2, "Meet the Overeating Styles" and the appendix, "The Evolution and Science Behind the Overeating Styles," for more about our research findings on the overeating styles.)

What You Eat, How You Eat, and Health

Alison's experience with Whole Person Integrative Eating, which we told you about earlier in this chapter, demonstrates how addressing the multidimensional WPIE *what*-and-*how*-to-eat elements of food and eating can be applied as a treatment plan for overcoming the overeating styles. Is it possible for others to overturn their overeating styles to enhance well-being? Researchers Erica Oberg and Ryan Bradley decided to find out.

When they applied the WPIE model and program to ten people with type 2 diabetes, they found that the *how* elements of WPIE (eating with positive emotions, mindfulness, appreciation, and loving regard and eating with others in a pleasant psychological and aesthetic atmosphere) lowered the A1C levels (a measure of blood-sugar levels) of research participants more than what they ate.[19,20]

Such findings prompted co-investigator Bradley to state, "How you eat appears to be as important, if not more important than what you eat."[20]

Oberg's study suggests that our WPIE model and program is a viable intervention for better health outcomes—in this case, for people with diabetes. At the same time, it has this powerful implication: overcoming *all* the overeating styles may bring better health outcomes than focusing on just one overeating style (which is typically *how much* and *what* a person eats). In other words, achieving successful health outcomes may depend on changing multiple eating behaviors, because our research reveals there are multiple reasons people overeat.

Improved Food Choices, Enhanced Eating Behaviors

Ultimately, our research on Whole Person Integrative Eating identifies the root causes of overeating and ensuing weight gain, while providing detailed insights into food choices and eating behaviors that can lead to overcoming overeating while enjoying food more.[3,7] Erica Oberg's study showed that replacing the overeating styles with WPIE-based eating behaviors—*how* people ate—lowered blood glucose levels for diabetics more than what they ate.[19,20]

And when researcher Erin Yaseen administered our "What's Your Overeating Style? Self-Assessment Quiz" to seventeen healthy, nonsmoking adults, ages eighteen to forty-nine years, her findings replicated our discovery about the link between the overeating styles, overeating, and being overweight.[3,7] Specifically, Yaseen found that those who overate and had the *highest* percentage of body fat scored especially high in the "Fast Foodism" and "Sensory Disregard" overeating styles. Conversely, those who followed the elements of our Whole Person Integrative Eating dietary lifestyle, meaning the *antidotes* to the overeating styles, had a lower percentage of body fat and overate less—especially in response to emotional stress *and* other "disinhibiting stimuli." Concludes Yaseen: "Evaluation of integrative eating may improve our understanding of behavioral contributors to obesity."[21]

Yet another key question about our Whole Person Integrative Eating program is this: can—and will—people adopt our integrative eating program and in turn improve their food choices and eating behaviors? To find out, I gave two one-hour lectures on Whole Person Integrative Eating and the seven overeating styles to seventy-five health-psychology students at San Francisco State University. The teaching sessions included having the students complete the "What's Your Overeating Style? Self-Assessment Quiz"[13] before the lectures and again six weeks afterward.

What we learned was this: two one-hour lectures—in addition to filling out our overeating styles self-assessment quiz before and after the lectures—were enough to help students improve on each of the overeating styles. Indeed, the students' overall integrative-eating scores improved by one full standard deviation six weeks after the lectures.

The changes in food choices (what they ate) and eating behaviors (how they ate) were significant (meaning not by chance) but moderate, and they were all in the same positive direction. A sampling: students made smarter food choices (for instance, less fried food and more fruits and veggies), and they made improvements in their eating behaviors (such as fewer emotional-eating episodes).[22]

Whole Person Integrative Eating: A Re-Visioning of Nutritional Health

A key takeaway from our research is this: Not only do the overeating styles identify and address *root reasons* many of us overeat and gain weight, our self-assessment quiz and ensuing research findings suggest that overeating and related weight gain is part of a complex web of more than food choices and how much people eat; it also includes the feelings, sensory experiences, and social behaviors linked to *how* people eat.

During the coaching sessions with Alison over the course of a year, after she identified her overeating styles, she discovered that in addition to awareness of what she was eating, "feeding" herself emotionally, spiritually, and socially (ergo, "whole person") each time she ate was also satisfying. And when she was nourished this way, she no longer needed to compensate with overeating and satiety. Alison's experience supports our research findings: Research participants who ate the most at the start of the six-week, eighteen-lesson, *Spirituality & Health* WPIE e-course enjoyed food the least. Yet once they learned to instinctively eat less food overall but choose more nourishing food, they enjoyed the experience of food and eating more.

The ancient-food-wisdom-based Whole Person Integrative Eating dietary lifestyle I tell you about in Part Two of this book is the antidote to each of the overeating styles.

Many investigators work in his or her own area of elements of Whole Person Integrative Eating, such as what to eat, emotional eating, mindfulness, social support, and so on. Surprisingly, there have yet to be studies on *all* of these optimal-eating interventions combined and its influence on weight.

Ultimately, the Whole Person Integrative Eating dietary lifestyle addresses the question: What would happen if, instead of focusing on each singular overeating style, people were empowered to change the multidimensional root causes of their overeating and ensuing weight gain by replacing them with the Whole Person Integrative Eating dietary lifestyle?

In other words, based on our research and on Alison's success with the Whole Person Integrative Eating dietary lifestyle, I am becoming increasingly convinced that it is not only what we eat that is contributing to overeating and the obesity pandemic, but also more "internal elements," such as emotional stress, negative emotions, spiritual emptiness, and social isolation—especially when we eat.

Essentially, the fundamental and recurring theme of this book is that treating overeating, overweight, and obesity through the lens of what and how much a person eats, without addressing the underlying emotional, mental, spiritual, and social causes, will provide only temporary weight loss, and the weight is likely to recur. Tackling the complex challenge of overeating and ensuing weight gain calls for an optimal-eating team, and we believe that each member of our Whole Person Integrative Eating program is part of the A team, because they work together as powerful antidotes to the overeating styles.

We are also posing this question: if our current knowledge about nutrition and our approach to food, eating, and weight aren't bringing the weight loss and health benefits many of us have hoped for, what, then, will work? We think the answer is our science-based, holistic, Whole Person Integrative Eating dietary lifestyle, which, at its core, nourishes you multidimensionally each time you eat.

But there's a caveat: changing your relationship to food and eating by learning Whole Person Integrative Eating is not a quick-fix, magical weight-loss program. Rather, it is a *lifetime practice*. Reaping the rewards depends on creating a new, whole person relationship to food, eating, and weight by practicing each element of WPIE each time you eat. Every chapter in this book gives you step-by-step guidelines to accomplish this.

The next chapter, "Meet the Overeating Styles 'Family': 7 Root Causes of Overeating," gives you the insights you need to understand the underlying reasons you may overeat and gain weight. It also offers detailed clues about the antidotes to the overeating styles, meaning the WPIE dietary lifestyle we tell you about in Part Two. Familiarizing yourself with the overeating styles is the first step toward creating a new recipe for weight-loss success. We wish you a wonderful journey.

CHAPTER 2

MEET THE OVEREATING STYLES "FAMILY": 7 ROOT CAUSES OF OVEREATING

Have you thought much about your relationship to food—the complex of eating behaviors, feelings, and thoughts you bring to the experience of food and eating? We have identified seven overeating styles linked to overeating and being overweight and obese. And the seven new overeating styles we've discovered include a complex of seventy-six food choices, emotions, and eating behaviors you bring to each meal.

If you're a food fretter, for instance, you may diet a lot and judge food as "good" or "bad." Perhaps you're a task snacker who eats while you watch TV, work, or drive. Are you an emotional eater who binges when you're bored, anxious, angry, or depressed? Is fast food, eaten alone and so quickly that you don't really taste it, your most-of-the-time fare? Or do you typically relate to food with all—or none—of the overeating styles?

The seven *statistically significant* overeating styles we discovered gave us new insights into many underlying reasons that so many of us overeat and gain weight.[1-3] We call these patterns of eating "styles" because they are sets of related food and eating behaviors that occur together consistently over time. The more you follow each overeating style—each of which is a new normal—the more likely you are to overeat, to feel badly about it, and to gain weight; conversely, the more you return to the culinary heritage that served humankind for millennia—the optimal-eating guidelines of our Whole Person Integrative Eating dietary lifestyle—the more likely you are to stop overeating and achieve normal weight . . . for life.

The seven overeating styles Larry and I tell you about in this chapter emerged when I took a step back to study what and how people had eaten for thousands of years[4] and then compared what I discovered to today's new-normal overeating styles. They are: Emotional Eating, Food Fretting, Fast Foodism, Sensory Disregard, Task Snacking, Unappetizing Atmosphere, and Solo Dining. (See "Appendix: The Evolution and Science Behind the Overeating Styles" for more about the science behind the overeating styles.)

Our discovery of new overeating styles provides illuminating nutritional insights into America's number-one health problem—the trilogy of overeating, overweight, and obesity—because we found that *not only are the seven overeating styles the new normal ways of eating, but they're all significantly and strongly linked to overeating. And five of the seven overeating styles are independently predictive of being overweight and obese (BMI).*[1]

We're excited to tell you about the overeating styles because they do more than provide practical insights into the personal reasons that you overeat and gain weight. What's especially meaningful about their discovery is this: The more our research participants[5,6] followed the new normal ways of eating, meaning the seven overeating styles we've identified, the more likely they were to overeat and be overweight and obese. *Conversely, the more they ate according to the ancient-food guidelines of our WPIE model and program* (which we tell you about in Part Two of this book)—*the less they overate and the more normal their weight.*[1] In other words, those who increasingly ate according to the perennial principles of WPIE after the online e-course we offered were the ones who lost the most weight.[1,6]

Another way of looking at the overeating styles is this: when you know your own overeating styles after taking the "What's Your Overeating Style? Self-Assessment Quiz"[7-9] in chapter 3, you're poised to practice the solutions we provide in Part Two of this book. The goal: to help you break the cycle of overeating and weight gain. The quiz in the next chapter will enable you to identify your own personal overeating styles—the areas you may want to pay attention to. But for now, meet the members of the overeating styles in the next section of this chapter.

Meet the Members:
The "Overeating Styles" Family

So you can familiarize yourself with each member of the overeating styles "family," here's a brief overview of each. We're presenting them to you in the order in which they predict overeating—from strongest to weakest.[1] As you look them over, consider whether you see yourself in any of them. (See the appendix, "The Evolution and Science Behind the Overeating Styles," for more about this.)

Emotional Eating

Most of us are familiar with the phrase "emotional eating," turning to comfort food to soothe negative feelings (such as depression, anxiety, or loneliness) but also to enhance joyous, celebratory emotions (in response, let's say, to a wedding, birthday, or promotion). If you often eat to manage your feelings and to self-soothe—in other words, for reasons other than hunger—it's likely you're an emotional eater.

Although all seven overeating styles are *statistically significant*, meaning all are key predictors that a person will overeat, the Emotional Eating overeating style is number one. In other words, negative emotions are the strongest indicators you'll turn to food to self-soothe and in turn overeat.

Some health professionals describe this overeating style as "compulsive overeating," "food addiction," or "self-medicating." No matter what it's called, many of us turn to food to relieve emotional tension because it works. For instance, did you know that carbohydrate-dense foods (such as cookies, cake, and bread) release a naturally occurring chemical messenger called serotonin? And that serotonin can calm and relax you? In this way, high-carb foods can soothe emotions that may be making you uncomfortable.

It may not come as a surprise that our research pinpointed Emotional Eating as the strongest predictor of overeating—and, therefore, the key contributor to weight gain. What you may find especially useful are the specific emotions we've identified—the family of emotions—that are strongly linked with the likelihood that you'll overeat.

Chapter 6, "Emotional Eating Rx: Positive Emotions," discusses Emotional Eating and the scientific strategies and positive feelings that can help you overcome overeating. We'll tell you about breakthrough brain-chemistry research that shows how turning to certain foods may mean you're self-medicating—which in turn may set off a binge in order to feel better. We shed light on the foods—and the specific nutrients in them—that can bust the blues, boost memory, cut carb cravings, and more. In essence, this chapter will give you the nutritional insights and tools you need to replace out-of-control Emotional Eating with the experience of choosing to eat with positive emotions and a healthy appetite. Chapter 13, "In Action: The WPIE Guided Meal

Meditation," gives you still more skills to turn out-of-control Emotional Eating into an intentional, WPIE, dine-with-pleasure experience.

Food Fretting

Good food, bad food. Legal food, illegal food. Sinful food, pure food. The food fretting overeating style is about being overly concerned about and focused on food, projecting moral judgment about what you or anyone else should or shouldn't eat, traditional dieting, thinking obsessively about the "right" way to eat, and basing your self-worth and that of others on what or how much is eaten. If you are often filled with such thoughts, you practice the food fretting style.

Below are some examples of Food Fretting "think." As you look them over, keep in mind that for some, calorie counting and awareness of unhealthful foods to avoid can serve as useful, helpful restraints to overeating. In other words, not all people who count calories or judge food are food fretters. The tipping point into Food Fretting is obsessing about the "best" way to eat and caloric intake.

Do you see yourself in any of the following examples of Food Fretting?

"I was good today," you may think when you've managed to avoid unhealthful foods, stick to your diet, and eat what you think you should.

"When my food cravings become powerful and I eat foods that are bad, I feel so guilty" is typical self-think for many food fretters.

"She should resist that sinful chocolate cake. Doesn't she have any willpower?" you might think as you watch someone eat what she "shouldn't."

Overcoming this eating style begins with recognizing such judgmental, fret-filled chatter about food and eating. Being honest with yourself will be challenging, since being critical and feeling anxious about food has become common in our culture. But the work you do to overcome this overeating style will be well worth the effort, because it will enable you to replace fret-filled self-think with empowering, WPIE-based smart-think.

In chapter 7, "Food Fretting Rx: Appreciate Food," we'll reveal the pitfalls of Food Fretting and the "think-filled" dimension of eating. As you'll see, a key underlying element of this weight-inducing overeating style is going on a traditional diet, then berating yourself if you go off the diet. Still, keep in mind that diets in and of themselves are not necessarily "bad." They can be a prescribed way of eating that is neutral, necessary, and helpful for many. It's the attitude behind the diet that makes it either helpful or a Food Fretting overeating style.

We will give you specific strategies for turning "disordered" thoughts and actions about food and eating into a whole person, nonjudgmental eating style so that you can appreciate food as a social, ceremonial, sensual pleasure—one that doesn't need to result in weight gain.

Fast Foodism

A donut or sugary cereal for breakfast; a McDonald's double burger with fries for lunch; and a supersized pizza, perhaps placed casually on the dining table in its cardboard box, for dinner—add several soft drinks throughout the day, and you have a profile of the fast-food cuisine that's typical for many Americans. Not surprisingly, this way of eating is strongly linked with overeating, overweight, and obesity—and it threatens more than your waistline.

As you'll discover, we qualify the solution with the phrase "as often as possible" to ensure that you don't interpret it as simply more dietary rules and regulations. Our intention is to help you think of what and how you eat as a spectrum rather than as all-or-nothing, black-or-white dietary dogma. To help you accomplish this, in chapter 8, "Fast Foodism Rx: Get Fresh," we show the link between fast foods and weight gain and the added ingredients that keep you from achieving your health goals. We demystify optimal eating and offer practical tips, exercises, and strategies to help you achieve and maintain a healthy relationship to food and well-being for a lifetime.

Sensory Disregard

How often do you focus on the aromas, colors, or flavors of food? Do you eat with your senses by appreciating the presentation, "tasting" the textures, or being grateful for the life-giving gift inherent in food? In our research, we found that those who ate the most actually enjoyed their food the least. Sensory Disregard is a powerful predictor of overeating and weight gain because if you're not enjoying your food—indeed, savoring it—you're likely to keep eating until you finally do feel a sense of satisfaction.

This may be the most overlooked aspect of overeating and ensuing weight gain. The problem is that many of us don't even know what it means to relate to food in a sensory way, let alone have a clue about how to convert to this way of eating that can make weight loss last. *Of all the overeating styles we've identified, sensory and spiritual disregard is associated with the largest number of food-related behaviors linked with overeating.*

Even if this overeating style is unfamiliar territory for you, it's likely a major contributor to overeating. If so, chapter 9, "Sensory Disregard Rx: Nourish Your Senses," will give you insights into the price your mind, body, and waistline pay if you typically make and eat meals without flavoring them with sensory and spiritual ingredients. You'll discover how to turn meals into palate-pleasing adventures that nourish both body and soul, for when you eat from the heart, you enjoy your meals in a far more meaningful way.

Task Snacking

Some call it "multitasking," the French call it "vagabond eating," and many in America think it's normal. However it's perceived, if you often eat while working by yourself in front of your computer, driving, watching TV, standing at the kitchen counter, shopping, or talking on the phone, it's likely that the Task Snacking overeating style is increasing your likelihood of overeating.

To counteract this overeating style, you'll discover how to rearrange your environment—both internally and externally. We'll show you how to work when you work, drive when you drive, and eat when you eat, rather than eating during other activities. You will find that making simple choices about eating mindfully can lead to big changes.

In chapter 10, "Task Snacking Rx: Mindfulness Eating," you'll discover the specific behaviors linked to Task Snacking that can contribute to weight gain. The antidote offered in the chapter will teach you how to break the cycle of merging eating with other activities. Eliminating Task Snacking completely isn't necessarily the goal; instead, we'll give you easy actions that you can take right now to cut down on your food-related multitasking, to pay attention to what you're eating, to enjoy your food, and in turn to reduce your overeating—and weight.

Unappetizing Atmosphere

You may find it surprising to learn that both the *psychological* and the *physical* atmospheres in which you eat can make a difference in whether you overeat. Turning around the Unappetizing Atmosphere overeating style will quickly improve the quality of your life by enhancing how you feel both physically and emotionally. It may even improve your relationships—with others as well as with food.

The psychological and physical dining aesthetics of your life can either contribute to satiety or lead to overeating. The psychological element refers to the emotions you experience within yourself and from others when you eat—feelings such as joy and happiness versus anger, fear, depression, and so on. The physical atmosphere includes your surroundings when you eat—at home, at the office, in restaurants, in your car, or at the homes of family and friends. Chapter 11, "Unappetizing Atmosphere Rx: Amiable Ambiance," will give you a repository of strategies for accessing the healing power inherent in a relaxing, aesthetically pleasing, and welcoming dining atmosphere.

Solo Dining

Chapter 12, "Solo Dining Rx: Share Fare," explains how dining by yourself can contribute to overeating and shows you the "ingredients" and skills you need to create enjoyable dining experiences with others.

To counteract the Solo Dining overeating style, we demonstrate how dining with others can be a balm for body, heart, and soul. You'll learn about the amazing healing possibilities of social dining that have been brought to light in scientific studies.

As your eating shifts from a "me" mentality to a "we" awareness—and, more and more, as you share food and the dining experience with others—you'll be taking yet another step toward fulfillment and weight loss.

These overeating styles offer insights into what we were hoping to find out when we started searching for the way of eating that had led to normal weight for so long and for what we're doing differently today. The new normal overeating styles may seem subtle on the surface, but they're all-encompassing in that not only does each one influence overeating and in turn weight, they differ drastically from what and how we ate for millennia.

In other words, since identifying these overeating styles, we've come to realize this simple fact about why so many of us struggle with weight: the more we veer away from the life-giving properties of food and the multidimensional ways in which it nourishes humankind (the essence of our Whole Person Integrative Eating program in Part Two of this book), the more we're likely to be overweight or obese, and the less we're likely to be able to lose weight and keep it off. Benefiting from our findings calls for reclaiming your food—and healthy-weight—heritage.

Overeating Styles: The New Normals

What do I mean when I state that the overeating styles are the new normal way of eating? If you take a closer look, you can see they are part of something that has changed in our relatively recent past (since about 1980, the increased prevalence of obesity began its precipitous rise), tipping overeating and obesity into a relentless—and worsening—epidemic that has made more than two-thirds of Americans either overweight or obese. Surely changes in our external and internal environments over the last few decades—what we consume, how much we eat, our physical activity, our sleep patterns, even our genes, an imbalanced microbiome, hormones, and an onslaught of toxic chemicals—are working together to make us overeat, feel bad about it, and gain weight.

Our own research has identified yet more changes in our relationship with food and eating over the last few decades that lead to overeating, overweight, and obesity: the new normal overeating styles. While the food choices and eating behaviors we have identified may seem familiar, comfortable, and normal for most of us, our research has revealed that our relationship to food and eating wasn't always like this. For centuries, wisdom traditions and cultural traditions provided whole person integrative eating guidelines that were the opposite of the overeating styles: consuming fresh food with others in a pleasant atmosphere and with positive emotions, mindfulness, gratitude, and loving regard.

Veering so far from what served humankind for millennia is having profound implications on our weight and well-being—physically, emotionally, spiritually, and socially. This is because the overeating styles' food choices and eating behaviors are relatively new in the evolution of humankind. We believe this means that our mind-body cannot metabolize adequately what I call "chemical cuisine"—fast, processed, and denatured food "products" (not food)—especially when we consume these products by ourselves, filled with negative emotions in stress-filled environments. Simply put, we're not meant to eat this way, and our mind-body is paying a big price with obesity and related chronic conditions.

We are excited to tell you about the overeating styles—in part because some very important ones have been overlooked by dieters, health professionals, and the diet industry, but mostly because our research findings have shown all seven to be statistically significant causes of overeating.[1] Without a doubt, each one is linked to overeating. At the same time, they identify specific food choices, emotions, and patterns of eating (eating behaviors) that predict, or result from, overeating and weight gain. In other words, all seven are part of an intricate web of food choices and eating behaviors that increase odds of overeating and becoming overweight or obese.

A New Recipe for Weight-Loss Success

The point is this: With the discovery of the overeating styles, we can look beyond conventional weight-loss wisdom by thinking of weight in terms of a family of food choices and eating behaviors you make each day. Unraveling all seventy-six elements of the overeating styles, identifying the ones that fit you, and then turning them around (we give you step-by-step guidelines for how to do this in Part Two, "The Whole Person Integrative Eating Dietary Lifestyle") is your best insurance for a lifetime of weight-loss success.

Our "What's Your Overeating Style? Self-Assessment Quiz"[7-9] in the next chapter gives you insights into your daily new-normal food choices, emotions, and eating behaviors that can lead to overeating and lead in turn to increased odds of being overweight and obese. By empowering you to understand not only what you eat but also the emotional, spiritual, and social dimensions of food and eating, the questionnaire is the first step in taking charge of your weight and well-being.

CHAPTER 3

WHAT'S YOUR OVEREATING STYLE? SELF-ASSESSMENT QUIZ

How are you eating now? Are you an Emotional Eater who binges when you're lonely, anxious, or depressed? Or is Food Fretting typical for you, replete with dieting and judging food as "good" or "bad"? Perhaps you're a Task Snacker who eats while you watch TV, work, or drive. Or maybe fast food eaten so quickly that you don't really taste it (Sensory Disregard) is your most-of-the-time fare. Then there's Solo Dining in an Unappetizing Atmosphere.

Based on our original research, these are the seven "new normal" overeating styles we've identified, which increase your odds of overeating and being overweight or obese.[1,2] In other words, the more overeating styles you engage in, the more you're at risk for overeating and gaining weight; conversely, when you take proactive steps each day to **stop the styles**, you up your odds of fulfilling your weight-loss potential.

Our "What's Your Overeating Style? Self-Assessment Quiz"[3-7] can help you discover the degree to which you are practicing—or not—each overeating style. Throughout the quiz, you'll discover how specific food choices you make work together with often-unexpected eating behaviors you typically practice that contribute to overeating and weight gain. In this way, the questionnaire will give you the insights you need to look beyond conventional weight-loss wisdom by thinking of weight in terms of a family of overeating behaviors and lifestyle choices.

Unraveling all the elements we introduce you to in the quiz and identifying the ones that apply to you is your best insurance for identifying your problem areas and then replacing them with the Whole Person Integrative Eating dietary lifestyle we tell you about in Part Two.

Stopping the Styles: A Lifetime Practice

Completing the profile prior to reading the rest of this book will give you baseline insights that you can use to measure improvements and changes in your overeating styles over time. The Whole Person Integrative Eating dietary lifestyle in Part Two will give you the proactive steps and insights you need to stop the styles and turn trouble areas into strengths. To reap the rewards, keep in mind that replacing the overeating styles with the Whole Person Integrative Eating dietary lifestyle is a lifetime *practice*. Over time, you'll be empowered to turn your personal team of overeating styles into an enjoyable, new relationship to food and eating that can help you make weight loss last.

Another benefit: we want you to know that the questionnaire has what researchers call "predictive validity," meaning each element within each overeating style is linked with overeating, overweight, and obesity.[1] In other words, our research on the overeating styles has verified that all seventy-six elements in the quiz carry weight (no pun intended!) in terms of the likelihood that a person will overeat and gain weight; they're not just questions Larry and I made up based on our personal beliefs, opinions, or observations.

Consider the profile to be a lighthouse that helps you get your bearings, a guide for determining your overeating-style food choices (*what* you eat) and eating behaviors (*how* you eat) so that you can choose the eating-style direction that will lead you naturally to weight-loss success.

Getting Started

Take our "What's Your Overeating Style? Self-Assessment Quiz" below to figure out the often-unexpected reasons you overeat and gain weight—and what you can do about it. After responding to the statements, you will discover your overeating style(s), learn about the elements that could be contributing to your overeating, and find ideas to guide your food choices and eating behaviors in the direction that can lead to weight loss, health, and healing.

As you tally your scores, keep in mind that the numbers you come up with are more than just numbers. Negative numbers provide nuggets of knowledge about behaviors that lead to weight gain, while positive scores highlight actions linked to weight loss.

Where Are You Now?

To find out, complete each overeating-style questionnaire. When you finish, you'll discover your Total Overeating Style Score. The interpretation about your score will give you the next steps you need to be a successful loser . . . for life.

DIRECTIONS

For Each Overeating Style:

Complete each overeating-style questionnaire below by checking the boxes that best represent your current eating style.

Some overeating-style sections have two parts. For these, score the top part by tallying all plus (+) numbers, and the bottom part by adding up the minus (−) numbers. Then subtract the minus total from the plus total and enter the result at the bottom of the overeating style.

At the bottom of each overeating-style profile, you'll find a key that tells you whether your score ranks as "excellent," "good," "satisfactory," or "needs improvement."

EMOTIONAL EATING
Overeating Style

For each question, check the box in the column that best represents your Emotional Eating dynamic.

	Never 0	Rarely +1	Some-times +2	Usually +3	Almost Always +4	Always +5
1. Before eating, I "check" my hunger level.	☐	☐	☐	☐	☐	☐
2. I eat only when I am hungry.	☐	☐	☐	☐	☐	☐

+
_____
Subtotal

	Never 0	Rarely -1	Some-times -2	Usually -3	Almost Always -4	Always -5
3. I overeat.	☐	☐	☐	☐	☐	☐
4. After eating, I feel stuffed.	☐	☐	☐	☐	☐	☐
5. I have food cravings.	☐	☐	☐	☐	☐	☐
6. I eat because I feel:						
depressed	☐	☐	☐	☐	☐	☐
sad	☐	☐	☐	☐	☐	☐
anxious	☐	☐	☐	☐	☐	☐
angry	☐	☐	☐	☐	☐	☐
frustrated	☐	☐	☐	☐	☐	☐
happy	☐	☐	☐	☐	☐	☐

-
_____
Subtotal

TOTAL EMOTIONAL EATING SCORE: **(+)** or **(-)** _____
Total

Emotional Eating Scoring Key

10 to -1	Excellent
-2 to -12	Good
-13 to -23	Satisfactory
-24 or less	Needs Improvement

FOOD FRETTING
Overeating Style

For each question, check the box in the column that best represents your Food Fretting dynamic.

	Never 0	Rarely -1	Some-times -2	Usually -3	Almost Always -4	Always -5
1. I feel anxious about the "best" way to eat.	☐	☐	☐	☐	☐	☐
2. I feel "good" or righteous when I eat what I think I "should."	☐	☐	☐	☐	☐	☐
3. When I overeat, I feel:						
bad	☐	☐	☐	☐	☐	☐
guilty	☐	☐	☐	☐	☐	☐
gluttonous	☐	☐	☐	☐	☐	☐
4. I judge others by what they eat	☐	☐	☐	☐	☐	☐
5. I try different diets.	☐	☐	☐	☐	☐	☐
6. I count calories, fat grams, etc.	☐	☐	☐	☐	☐	☐
7. I obsess about food.	☐	☐	☐	☐	☐	☐

TOTAL FOOD FRETTING SCORE:

-_____
Total

Food Fretting Scoring Key

0 to -7	Excellent
-8 to -14	Good
-15 to -21	Satisfactory
-22 or less	Needs Improvement

FAST FOODISM
Overeating Style

For each question, check the box in the column that best represents your Fast Foodism dynamic.

	Never	Rarely	Some-times	Usually	Almost Always	Always
	0	+1	+2	+3	+4	+5
1. I eat fresh:						
fruits	☐	☐	☐	☐	☐	☐
vegetables	☐	☐	☐	☐	☐	☐
whole grains	☐	☐	☐	☐	☐	☐
legumes	☐	☐	☐	☐	☐	☐
nuts	☐	☐	☐	☐	☐	☐
seeds (e.g., sunflower, flax)	☐	☐	☐	☐	☐	☐
2. I eat meals that are homemade.	☐	☐	☐	☐	☐	☐

+ _____

Subtotal

	Never	Rarely	Some-times	Usually	Almost Always	Always
	0	-1	-2	-3	-4	-5
3. I eat food that is:						
fast (such as McDonald's)	☐	☐	☐	☐	☐	☐
processed (canned, packaged)	☐	☐	☐	☐	☐	☐
prepared (deli, takeout)	☐	☐	☐	☐	☐	☐
sweet (donuts, muffins)	☐	☐	☐	☐	☐	☐
fried (potato chips, chicken)	☐	☐	☐	☐	☐	☐

- _____

Subtotal

TOTAL FAST FOODISM SCORE: **(+) or (-)**   _____

Total

Fast Foodism Scoring Key

35 to 23	Excellent
22 to 11	Good
10 to -1	Satisfactory
-2 or less	Needs Improvement

SENSORY DISREGARD
Overeating Style

For each question, check the box in the column that best represents your Sensory Disregard dynamic.

	Never 0	Rarely +1	Some- times +2	Usually +3	Almost Always +4	Always +5
1. I plan and prepare meals:						
with care	☐	☐	☐	☐	☐	☐
with appreciation	☐	☐	☐	☐	☐	☐
2. While dining, I consider my surroundings.	☐	☐	☐	☐	☐	☐
3. I express gratitude for food through prayer, blessings, heartfelt thankfulness.	☐	☐	☐	☐	☐	☐
4. I honor the mystery of life in food.	☐	☐	☐	☐	☐	☐
5. Before and during eating, I focus on the food's:						
color	☐	☐	☐	☐	☐	☐
aroma	☐	☐	☐	☐	☐	☐
portion size	☐	☐	☐	☐	☐	☐
flavor(s)	☐	☐	☐	☐	☐	☐
6. I "eat" with my senses by:						
appreciating the presentation	☐	☐	☐	☐	☐	☐
tasting textures	☐	☐	☐	☐	☐	☐
savoring scents	☐	☐	☐	☐	☐	☐
7. I focus solely on food and the experience of dining.	☐	☐	☐	☐	☐	☐
8. I appreciate the web of humanity (farmers, grocers) surrounding food.	☐	☐	☐	☐	☐	☐
9. I consider the elements of nature that create food.	☐	☐	☐	☐	☐	☐
10. I eat with loving regard for food.	☐	☐	☐	☐	☐	☐
11. After eating, I:						
savor the moment	☐	☐	☐	☐	☐	☐
reflect on the meal	☐	☐	☐	☐	☐	☐

TOTAL SENSORY DISREGARD SCORE: + _____

Total

Sensory Disregard Scoring Key

72 to 90	Excellent
54 to 71	Good
53 to 36	Satisfactory
35 or less	Needs Improvement

TASK SNACKING
Overeating Style

For each question, check the box in the column that best represents your Task Snacking dynamic.

	Never	Rarely	Some-times	Usually	Almost Always	Always
	0	-1	-2	-3	-4	-5
1. When I eat, I am...						
walking, rushing somewhere	☐	☐	☐	☐	☐	☐
at my desk at work	☐	☐	☐	☐	☐	☐
in my car	☐	☐	☐	☐	☐	☐
at my computer	☐	☐	☐	☐	☐	☐
talking on the phone	☐	☐	☐	☐	☐	☐
driving	☐	☐	☐	☐	☐	☐

TOTAL TASK SNACKING SCORE: - _____

Total

Task-Snacking Scoring Key

0 to - 6	Excellent
-7 to -12	Good
-13 to -17	Satisfactory
-18 or less	Needs Improvement

UNAPPETIZING ATMOSPHERE
Overeating Style

For each question, check the box in the column that best represents your Unappetizing Atmosphere dynamic.

	Never	Rarely	Some-times	Usually	Almost Always	Always
	0	+1	+2	+3	+4	+5
1. The social atmosphere in which I prepare food is:						
serene	☐	☐	☐	☐	☐	☐
pleasing	☐	☐	☐	☐	☐	☐
fun	☐	☐	☐	☐	☐	☐
2. After eating, I feel:						
relaxed	☐	☐	☐	☐	☐	☐
calm	☐	☐	☐	☐	☐	☐
alert	☐	☐	☐	☐	☐	☐

+ _____

Subtotal

	Never	Rarely	Some-times	Usually	Almost Always	Always
	0	-1	-2	-3	-4	-5
3. The social atmosphere in which I prepare food is:						
hectic	☐	☐	☐	☐	☐	☐
tense	☐	☐	☐	☐	☐	☐

- _____

Subtotal

TOTAL UNAPPETIZING ATMOSPHERE SCORE: **(+)** or **(-)** _____

Total

Unappetizing Atmosphere Scoring Key

30 to 22	Excellent
21 to 14	Good
13 to 6	Satisfactory
5 or less	Needs Improvement

SOLO DINING
Overeating Style

For each question, check every box in the column that best represents your Solo Dining dynamic.

	Never 0	Rarely +1	Some-times +2	Usually +3	Almost Always +4	Always +5
1. I eat with:						
friends	☐	☐	☐	☐	☐	☐
family members	☐	☐	☐	☐	☐	☐
2. I eat at home at the dining table.	☐	☐	☐	☐	☐	☐
3. I enjoy preparing meals for friends.	☐	☐	☐	☐	☐	☐
4. I enjoy holiday feasts with others.	☐	☐	☐	☐	☐	☐
5. I celebrate special occasions with others with festive foods.	☐	☐	☐	☐	☐	☐
6. I prepare and share special meals for friends and family.	☐	☐	☐	☐	☐	☐
7. When eating alone, I often think about special people in my life, or memorable meals I've enjoyed with others.	☐	☐	☐	☐	☐	☐

+ _____

Subtotal

	Never 0	Rarely -1	Some-times -2	Usually -3	Almost Always -4	Always -5
8. I eat alone.	☐	☐	☐	☐	☐	☐
9. I plan "secret" overeating sessions.	☐	☐	☐	☐	☐	☐
10. I dine with others, then, afterward, binge by myself.	☐	☐	☐	☐	☐	☐
11. I stand at the counter while eating.	☐	☐	☐	☐	☐	☐

- _____

Subtotal

TOTAL SOLO DINING SCORE: **(+)** or **(-)** _____

Total

Solo Dining Scoring Key

40 to 28	Excellent
27 to 16	Good
15 to 4	Satisfactory
3 or less	Needs Improvement

YOUR TOTAL SCORE

Tallying Your Total Overeating-Style Score

1. Enter the positive scores for each of the seven eating styles in the "Positive Subtotals" column.

2. Enter the negative scores for each of the seven eating styles in the "Negative Subtotals" column.

3. For your total score, subtract the negative total from the positive total.

Overeating Style	Positive Subtotals	Negative Subtotals
Emotional Eating	_____	_____
Food Fretting	_____	_____
Fast Foodism	_____	_____
Sensory Disregard	_____	_____
Task Snacking	_____	_____
Unappetizing Atmosphere	_____	_____
Solo Dining	_____	_____

Positive Total _____ **Negative Total** _____

TOTAL OVEREATING STYLE SCORE: _____

INTERPRETING YOUR SCORE

131 or More: Excellent

Congratulations! The "excellent" level is comparable to an A+. Your relationship with food is mostly satisfying and gratifying—and you enjoy food and eating most of the time. Both what and how you eat are beneficial to your weight, your overall health, and your quality of life.

A score of "excellent" suggests that the overeating styles aren't typical for you, and that you are already practicing many of the Whole Person Integrative Eating solutions that make weight loss last. For still more benefits, look over your answers for each overeating style and target additional changes you could make to optimize your relationship to food even more. Our antidotes to the overeating styles in Part Two of this book can give you still more optimal-eating ideas.

130 to 57: Good

You're doing fairly well! The "good" level gives you a grade between A and B+. What you eat, how you eat, and with whom you eat are typically positive and beneficial. You eat optimally sometimes; when you're not able to—or choose not to—you let it go.

To improve your relationship to food and eating, look over your answers and decide whether there are changes you'd like to make to bring you closer to Whole Person Integrative Eating. Then become familiar with the overeating styles—particularly those to which you seem to have some resistance. Become familiar with the antidotes to the overeating styles in Part Two of this book.

56 to -14: Satisfactory

Food and eating are often issues for you. The way you typically eat is comparable to a grade between B and C. You may have some confusion about what and how to eat optimally, or overcoming your overeating style(s) hasn't been a priority so far. Your relationship to food and eating is fairly typical, which leaves lots of room for making beneficial changes.

A score of "satisfactory" suggests that you may find it challenging to practice many of the solutions to the overeating styles that we tell you about in Part Two of this book. Look over your answers for each overeating style to target specific changes you'd like to make to lead you closer to Whole Person Integrative Eating. Then "meet" the overeating styles—particularly those to which you seem to have some resistance—and look over the chapters in Part Two for more helpful suggestions about the overeating styles you would like to address.

-15 or Below: Needs Improvement

Your overall eating style is far from optimal. Decide whether you want to take steps toward improving your relationship with food. To help you do this, first read chapter 4, "Are You Really Ready to Lose Weight?," for insights into launching your successful loser strategies. Once you're clear about wanting to make changes, look over the questions for—and your answers to—each overeating style in this quiz to target specific changes you'd like to make.

A score of "needs improvement" suggests that you would benefit greatly by learning about and then living the practical, step-by-step solutions we reveal throughout this book. Remember, small steps can lead to big benefits. A good place to start: "meet" the overeating styles in chapter 2, then discover the proactive steps you can take to overcome them in Part Two.

Overcoming the Overeating Styles

Whatever your findings from our overeating-styles questionnaire, it's possible for you to use the results to manage your overeating and weight. How? By practicing and living the solutions to the seven overeating styles we tell you about in Part Two, so that body, mind, and soul are nourished each time you eat. Be aware, though, that what *you* contribute is at least as important as the insights and information we provide. There are three requisites for you to be successful: 1) a firm commitment to changing your approach to food and eating; 2) a willingness to take the necessary time to make beneficial changes; 3) and a commitment to a heartfelt regard for food and all food-related activities.

In the following chapter, "Are You Really Ready to Lose Weight?," we'll introduce you to profound, practical, and pragmatic guidelines—the additional "ingredients" you need—to reap the rewards of the Whole Person Integrative Eating dietary lifestyle we tell you about in Part Two. With insights into your readiness to attain and maintain weight loss, you'll be empowered to overcome your own overeating styles and increase your chances of making weight loss last.

CHAPTER 4

ARE YOU REALLY READY TO LOSE WEIGHT?

Remember Alison, whom we told you about in chapter 1? Like millions of us, she has struggled with being obese for decades. When Alison felt overwhelmed and frustrated with her weight, she would think, "I've got to do something about this. It's time to diet." Then *WOOSH!* She would do what most of us do: Pick the latest diet du jour, believing this time would be different. She would follow the strict guidelines, lose weight, and be slim. But would she stay slim? Well . . . it hadn't happened . . . yet. When food cravings overwhelmed her, she would give in to them . . . and gain back the weight she had lost . . . and often more.

Scientific studies have reminded us, over and over, that diets don't work. Yet, like Alison, most continue to jump onto the restrict-what-you-eat diet bandwagon as soon as I-can't-take-this-weight-anymore "think" strikes. What can you do differently to stop going from panic and frustration to traditional dieting that doesn't work? To instead nourish yourself with the Whole Person Integrative Eating dietary lifestyle . . . for life? In other words, what can you do to discover if you're really ready to lose weight . . . and keep it off? Let's find out.

A Successful Loser Secret?
Meet the 5 Stages of Change

Two decades ago, psychologists James Prochaska and Carlo DiClemente developed a pioneering model for how people change eating and other lifestyle habits, such as smoking, stress management, and physical activity.[1-7]

The "five stages of change" they discovered have special significance for the millions who struggle with weight, because not only do the stages identify what it takes to make changes that stick, but the psychologists' step-by-step process reveals that true change requires an experiential, internal shift in a person's attitudes and perception—indeed, in their way of being.

This means that if you work your way through each of the stages, you *strongly* up your odds of losing weight and keeping it off. But the converse is also true: if you don't take the time to familiarize yourself with each of the changes and then "graduate" from each stage, you're more likely to fail to make lasting change . . . in what you eat, how you eat, and what you weigh.

Achieving True Transformation

What may be of special interest about the stages of change to the many millions who go on diets—and then gain back more weight than they lost—is this fascinating factoid: the stages reveal that changing for the long term often involves setbacks, but with repeated efforts the chances for success increase. In other words, making changes in your relationship to food so that you lose weight and keep it off is not a black-or-white, all-or-nothing decision. Rather, the stages of change reveal it's a process, and "failure" isn't really failure (unless you quit); it's actually part of a cycle that leads to success if, as the song goes, you pick yourself up, brush yourself off, and start all over again (reworking the stages helps a lot).

Indeed, Prochaska and DiClemente posit that to achieve lasting change, it's quite normal to need to make more than one attempt.[1] Their research also revealed that a large part of weight-loss success depends on working your way through the stages of change to discover if you're really, really ready to lose weight and keep it off. Or, conversely, is it something you "should" do or "want" to do, but in reality, you are really not ready for true transformation? Wending your way through the stages of change can help you answer such questions—which are pivotal to weight-loss success for the long term.

This is Also Pivotal to Weight-Loss Success

The mistake most of us make when we think of losing weight by "going on a diet" is being ignorant about where we are in the stages-of-change cycle. Once you know which stage you're in, you can wisely and thoughtfully progress to the next stage. By not jumping ahead to a stage for which you may not be ready (such as taking action and going on a diet before doing appropriate planning to remove obstacles), you lower the odds of slipping back into old eating habits. In other words, the stages of change up your odds of being a successful loser by giving you insights into how to change, as well as specific strategies for how you can best help yourself achieve true transformation in your relationship to food, eating, and weight.

Meet the Stages-of-Change Cycle

Are you really ready to lose weight, or do you just want to? Spend time with the stages, and you'll know the answer. Here they are: pre-contemplation, contemplation, preparation, action, maintenance, and relapse. Familiarize yourself with the stages, then take the time to identify the stage you're in right now. You'll know if and when you are ready to change when you understand the stage you're in and stay with that stage until you're truly, deep-down ready to move on to the contemplation stage or the action stage. Empowered by these self-insights, you'll be poised to turn the defeatism of traditional dieting upside down.

Pre-contemplation. This is a kind of precursor to the four other, more formal stages that empower you to change your food choices, eating behaviors, and weight. You're in the pre-contemplation stage if you're not yet interested in changing your food and eating habits ("This is the way I am; I'm big-boned"), if you're not concerned about being overweight ("Most Americans are overweight; I fit right in"), or if you don't recognize that you have a problem with food or weight ("It's society's problem, not mine"). You may also be ignorant of health risks linked with overweight or obesity and instead blame your weight on biology, metabolism, or genes inherited from your parents. You're not too open to advice, and you're not yet contemplating change.

Contemplation. The contemplation stage is the stage Alison was in when she contacted me. She was thinking about changing what and how she ate, and she was kind of easing into changing—perhaps she would get to it tomorrow or sometime in the next few months. At this stage, you may have some ambivalence, because considering a change in lifelong food and eating habits can be a life-altering decision. As you progress through contemplation, you will come to a decision about your next step.

Preparation (an unofficial but important stage). Most of us skip the preparation stage and immediately go from contemplation ("I should go on a diet") to taking action (dieting). I believe skipping this stage is why most of us fail at losing weight and keeping it off. Because too many people skip this stage, Alison and I spent a lot of time in this state, considering the benefits she was getting out of her current way of eating (the pros), and what she found frustrating and unacceptable (the cons).

In other words, in the preparation stage—prior to taking action and going on a diet—you're getting in touch with the downside (the cons) of the current way you relate to food, eating, and weight; at the same time, you're considering, organizing, and planning the benefits (the pros) of changing your relationship to food. If you're in this stage, you've decided to make a change; you've shifted from "I ought to" to "I'm going to." Making changes in your food choices and overeating styles (see chapter 2, "Meet the Overeating Styles 'Family': 7 Root Causes of Overeating" for more about this) is just around the corner; you're planning to do it within the next month.

To prepare for success when you make your shift into the next action stage, first weigh the pros and cons of your current relationship to food and eating. What is the *downside* to what and how you are currently eating? What are the *benefits* you'll receive by changing your relationship to food? What's working well for you? What exactly needs to change? What is keeping you from making changes? After you've thought through the pros and cons, it's time to create your plan of action.

Action. During the preparation stage, you identified obstacles (the cons) to making changes as well as strengths (the pros) you bring with you along the journey. You have entered the action stage when you've prepared yourself for change and created specific steps.

Prior to taking action and making changes in what and how she ate, Alison told me she enjoyed fresh, flavor-filled food that was beautifully presented. So we talked about where she would get this kind of food and where she would eat it.

Now she was motivated and ready to implement the plan of action she had been thinking about for the past weeks—actually, months. She was ready to put into action the Whole Person Integrative Eating Dietary Lifestyle we tell you about in Part Two. When we started working together, Alison had filled out the "What's Your Overeating Style? Self-Assessment Quiz," so we both were familiar with the over-eating styles that were challenging for her. With such insights, Alison decided she would begin with the antidote to the Unappetizing Atmosphere overeating style: she would create an "Amiable Ambiance" in her home: a charming dining nook replete with aesthetically pleasing place mats and dishes. Not only was Alison clear about what she wanted to achieve and how she was going to go about it, but she was actually ready to do it, be it, and live it.

Maintenance. Maintaining optimal food choices, eating behaviors, and weight loss calls for progressing through the previous stages until they become habitual. Keep in mind that it typically takes months to change a habit (at least two months; sometimes as much as eight months) and to achieve lasting change. This may be a good time to weigh the benefits and obstacles you identified in the preparation stage and to make changes accordingly. (To up your odds of success, please see Part Three, "Whole Person Integrative Eating Recipes," for menu plans and recipes.)

Relapse. The stages of change aren't an all-or-none proposition (unlike most approaches to traditional dieting); rather, as with our Whole Person Integrative Eating dietary lifestyle, they're a *process*, a *practice*, a *journey*—with guidelines for transitioning from the Food Fretting overeating style and yo-yo dieting to lasting change.

Throughout the process, realize that it's common to return to what's familiar and comfortable, even though it may not be what you want or what's good for you. Be aware that many of us will relapse and return to prior eating habits and food choices for a short or long time. This isn't the time to get discouraged and give up. Instead, go back over the stages and plan how to overcome the obstacle that got in your way (see our epilogue for more insights into overcoming obstacles). When you've done this, return to the action stage. Be compassionate with yourself, and repeat each of the stages until the action stage becomes second nature.[2]

The key point is this: if and when you find you're in the "Relapse" stage, you haven't failed. This stage is normal and is to be expected! If relapse occurs, review the pros and cons you discovered in the preparation stage, then return to your Whole Person Integrative Eating dietary lifestyle. Remember, it's a lifetime *practice*; it's not something you go on, then off again.

From Dieting . . . to Self-Reflection . . . to Success

Food choices (such as fast, processed junk food versus fresh, whole food) and eating-related behaviors (such as overeating) are deeply instilled habits that, for most of us, are hard to change—*unless you find out where you are in the stages-of-change model and then progress through each stage.* Here's the tip you need to use the stages to strongly up your odds of attaining and maintaining weight loss:

Are You Really Ready to Lose Weight?

Reset your **intention** from "going on a diet" to "befriending" the stages of change so you can transform your relationship to food, eating, and weight in a deep, profound way. (Please see the "A 'Way of Life,' Not a Diet" section in chapter 5, "What's a Dietary Lifestyle, Anyway? (Hint: Overeating Styles Rx)" for more about this.)

In other words, losing weight and keeping it off calls for true transformation—discovering how to nourish yourself on a meaningful, experiential, personal level. With this in mind, please read this entire chapter again to see how you can apply the stages of change to your life and relationship to food and eating. Really "get it." And be sure to take time to do the "preparation" self-reflection it takes to jump off the dieting treadmill and instead be a successful loser. The challenge: to decide if you're really ready to lose weight . . . for life.

Once you've gleaned insights from the stages of change in this chapter, you're poised to reap the rewards of the Whole Person Integrative Eating dietary lifestyle we tell you about in Part Two, the next section of this book. We created this how-to section to empower you to overcome any or all the overeating styles.

As you'll see, each chapter is resplendent with scientific studies and stories that support each WPIE guideline. And the practical tips, tools, skills, and strategies in each WPIE chapter show you how to transform your overeating style's relationship to food, eating, and weight, and in the process find true nourishment. We wish you a wonderful Whole Person Integrative Eating journey.

PART TWO

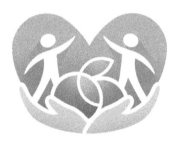

The Whole Person Integrative Eating Dietary Lifestyle

CHAPTER 5

WHAT'S A DIETARY LIFESTYLE, ANYWAY? (HINT: OVEREATING STYLES Rx)

What if it were possible that what you eat and how you eat could help you lose weight, keep it off, and overcome other diet-related conditions such as heart disease, diabetes, and high blood pressure? And what if you were able to achieve such health and healing by returning to your food roots—going back to the Whole Person Integrative Eating dietary lifestyle we've been telling you about throughout this book—a relationship to food and eating that nourished humankind physically, emotionally, spiritually, and socially for millennia? In other words, might returning to your food roots help you turn the tide of today's pandemic of diet-related chronic conditions?

Sculpture artist Roxanne Swentzell—whose carvings are featured in the Smithsonian in Washington, D.C., and in her Tower Gallery in Pojoaque, New Mexico, among other venues—decided to find out if returning to her ancestral diet would help her and her native family and friends heal. A descendant of the Pueblo peoples of New Mexico, Swentzell decided to launch a study to see if consuming the original foods of her people would turn the tide of the chronic conditions that threatened the health of both herself and many of her people.

Swentzell's journey back to her ancestral diet began in 2012 when she and her family and friends realized they were all facing a multitude of health problems. Swentzell was overweight and had high cholesterol, high blood pressure, and other diet-related health problems; her eight-year-old grandson was diagnosed with prediabetes; her son was obese with heart disease; and other ancestors had diabetes and were battling obesity, autoimmune diseases, chronic fatigue, and depression. Porter, Swentzell's son, wondered if they would be healthier if they ate the way their ancestors did instead of eating today's standard American diet (SAD) of fast, processed, denatured food.[1-3]

The question Swentzell asked was this: What would happen if we—Native American Pueblo people—ate like our ancestors in to-day's time? The "we" Swentzell is referring to is her tribe, the San-ta Clara Pueblo people, who have lived in the Santa Clara Pueblo (Kha'p'oo Owinge, meaning *Valley of the Wild Roses*), twenty-four miles north of Santa Fe, New Mexico, since about 1550. Puebloans and descendants of the original Spanish settlers, who had also lived in this area for hundreds of years, would be included in Swentzell's "return-to-our-food-roots" culinary experiment.

The first step: deciding who would participate in the project and deciding the time period. After Swentzell and thirteen friends and family members from pueblos across northern New Mexico agreed to go back to their basic, pre-European foods, they committed to try out their new ancient diet for three months.

Step two: the "research participants" turned their food odyssey into an informal scientific study by recording starting weight and get-ting basic blood work that included cholesterol and blood-sugar levels.

Step three: figuring out what their Santa Clara Pueblo ancestors ate circa 1590. The conclusion: before the Spanish influenced their diet, typical indigenous fare was wild game (such as birds, elk, deer, and buffalo); fish; wild vegetables (beans, corn, squash—called "the three sisters"—spinach, and more); and fruit, especially small, sweet strawberries. All "new normal," post-European, processed food prod-ucts would be eliminated, including sugar, alcohol, wheat and white flour, beef, and chicken. Swentzell realized their bodies couldn't han-dle processed food very well.

The findings: Twelve weeks after eating their origins diet, all fourteen members of the Santa Clara Pueblo group had their blood tested again. The health status of all participants improved . . . a lot. Writes Grand Canyon Trust's Native American Program Man-ager Deon Ben about Swentzell's new health status: "After years of struggling with what her doctor had diagnosed as genetic high blood pressure . . . after just three months of eating Native foods, her condition was gone."[3] And it gets better. Swentzell had lost fif-teen pounds, and her cholesterol levels had normalized too. And all other participants had similar successes: Her son lost fifty pounds during this time (he has since attained and maintained a weight loss of ninety pounds). All lost weight, think better, have more energy, and normalized many biomarkers.

And all these healing mind-body benefits happened because Swentzell and her fellow ancestors returned to their food roots—to the foods their ancestors ate for centuries—to a *dietary lifestyle* they reclaimed (and still make) as their own.

Now, several years later, this kind of eating has become a way of life for Swentzell. Today, there's no refrigerator in Swentzell's kitchen. After all, her ancestors from the Santa Clara Pueblo didn't refrigerate food. She continues to follow the original ancestral food ways of the Pueblo peoples, which means eating crops of fresh food, grown or captured nearby, that don't need to be kept cold. Her diet is a wide variety of fruits, vegetables, whole grains, legumes, nuts, seeds, and chemical-free meat, fowl, and fish. Recipes include such indigenous fare as buffalo tamales, blue-corn cakes, and rabbit stew and delicacies ranging from prickly pear and grasshoppers to marrowbone butter.[1-4]

As ideal as it is, surely the indigenous dietary lifestyle Roxanne follows is an extreme example of returning to one's "food roots." For most of us, such a pure return is not practical. Still, the point is this: returning to a dietary lifestyle of fresh, whole foods—based on foods our ancestors ate—brings health and healing. And it makes meals personal and meaningful—rather than being a directive from an "expert" about what you *should* eat.

A "Way of Life," Not a Diet

When Swentzell and her ancestors reclaimed (lived?) their traditional diet, they were more in tune with the time of Greek physician Hippocrates (460–370 B.C.) and the wisdom traditions (please see the introduction, "Ancient Food Wisdom Meets Modern Nutritional Science," for more about this). It was during this time in ancient Greece that the word *diet* (*diaita*) meant an entire "way of life" that encompassed food, drink, and lifestyle. Indeed, over the centuries, *diet* evolved from its original ancient meaning of "way of life" to reflect the Old French (*diete*) Middle English definition of "restricting oneself to small amounts or special kinds of food; or to eat sparingly to lose weight, or for medical reasons" (familiar, isn't it?).[5,6] This is quite a contrast to today's meaning of the word *diet*, which most of us connect to the idea of deprivation and restriction.

When Swentzell and her ancestors reconnected to their food origins, instead of approaching food, eating, weight, and well-being with today's sense of dread, worry, and anxiety and going on a diet, they connected to food based on its original meaning: a way of living that could help them achieve optimal weight and other health benefits. But their odyssey also helped them to accomplish even more, for by continuing their new old way of eating, they turned their newfound relationship to their ancestral diet into a dietary lifestyle that nourished them not only physically but also emotionally, spiritually, and socially. Such a comprehensive relationship to food and eating is the basis of the Whole Person Integrative Eating program we're telling you about in this book.

Whole Person Integrative Eating: A Re-Visioning of Nutritional Health

Only a few decades ago, conventional nutrition viewed the body as a machine whose weight was determined by a calories-in, calories-out formula. Most health professionals were taught the mind and body were separate and independent from each other and that biochemical reactions and genes determined our health status and weight.

With paradigm-shifting medical discoveries about the human genome, epigenetics, and the microbiome and its mind-body link in the twenty-first century, the scientific community's view of the influence of food on health and healing is evolving quickly. Add the evolution of new food-and-diet-based medical specialties such as Dean Ornish, M.D.'s lifestyle medicine[7-9] and Jeffrey Bland, Ph.D.'s functional medicine[10]—and many researchers are arriving at a radically different understanding about the power of food to reset your genes, your microbiome, and your mind-body for either wellness or illness.

With our discovery of the overeating styles and our Whole Person Integrative Eating dietary lifestyle, we believe that our research may also contribute to a re-visioning of the new nutrition "think" that's been emerging in the twenty-first century. This is because our studies on the seven overeating styles we have identified reveal a defined pattern of daily food choices and eating behaviors practiced by most Americans that lead to their overeating, overweight, and obesity.

What's of special interest about the discovery of the overeating styles is that they apply to both males and females, for all ages and education levels, and for four ethnicities (Caucasian, Hispanic, African American, Native American).[11] This means that each overeating style is a clearly defined, separate pattern of eating behaviors that are so consistent, they can justifiably be called independent overeating styles.

The takeaway: our research establishes the Whole Person Integrative Eating dietary lifestyle we tell you about in Part Two as more than mere recommendations and guidelines. Rather, the WPIE program and our validated "What's Your Overeating Style? Self-Assessment Quiz" are substantive, practical, scientifically sound whole-person tools that, by raising awareness about what and how a person eats, offer the antidotes to the overeating styles.

Given our whole-person findings about the influence of food and eating on biological, psychological, spiritual, and social well-being, we are positing that simpler approaches fail in terms of long-term weight-loss maintenance because they likely address only what to eat or just one overeating style, such as Emotional Eating. In other words, an oversimplified approach ignores the web of multidimensional, inter-related thoughts, feelings, beliefs, food choices, and eating behaviors that influence overeating, overweight, and obesity. In turn, we believe that ignoring these factors could up the odds of relapse, meaning, you're more likely to return to your usual way of eating and the ensuing weight gain that goes along with it.

Ultimately, we think that the discovery of the overeating styles—and their antidote, our Whole Person Integrative Eating dietary lifestyle—provides a paradigm-shifting framework for addressing what, how, and why Americans overeat and gain weight.[11] At the same time, our validated "What's Your Overeating Style? Self-Assessment Quiz"[12,13] reveals and assesses the specific overeating styles and re-lated behaviors. After filling out the overeating styles quiz, it is easy to see the overeating styles that are most problematic for a person as well as the microelements that are especially challenging within each overeating style.

In turn, people can make immediate decisions about the overeat-ing style(s) and specific eating behaviors that need attention. The an-tidote? Our Whole Person Integrative Eating model and program, which provides step-by-step guidelines for replacing each overeating style with scientifically sound strategies for overcoming overeating and reducing odds of overweight and obesity.

The takeaway: by defining and expanding our knowledge and un-derstanding about why we overeat and what we can do about it, we believe our discovery of the overeating styles and their antidote, our Whole Person Integrative Eating model and program, is a "family" of both the external and visible (what you eat and with whom you eat), and the internal and invisible (eating with positive emotions, mind-fulness, gratitude, and loving regard) "ingredients" that influence physical, emotional, spiritual, and social well-being (ergo, "whole person") and ultimately, your weight and mind-body well-being.[11] We are presenting it as a sustainable dietary lifestyle, a lifetime practice, and a re-visioning of nutritional health that may help people overcome overeating, overweight, and obesity.

Definition: Whole Person Integrative Eating

We define Whole Person Integrative Eating as a multidimensional dietary lifestyle: a holistic, multidimensional approach to food and eating that involves research, prevention, treatment, and reversal of overeating, overweight, and obesity and other food-related chronic conditions.[14] At the same time, WPIE integrates the four facets of food discussed in chapter 1: Biological Nutrition (food and physical health), Psychological Nutrition (food and feelings), Spiritual Nutrition (eating with mindfulness, appreciation, and loving regard), and Social Nutrition (eating with others in pleasant psychological and aesthetic atmospheres), with an emphasis on food choices (what one eats), emotions (why one eats), and eating behaviors (how one eats).

Another key concept of WPIE is this: WPIE is a lifetime practice designed to cultivate 1) awareness of a whole-person way of relating to food and eating 2) and self-regulation of what, why, how, where, and with whom one eats. In this way, we believe that WPIE can be a lifetime practice that addresses the widening split between today's conventional external focus on food and eating (such as the new normal of "eating by number"—counting calories, carbs, fat grams, etc.) and a lack of attention to the inner experience of eating (with positive emotions, mindfulness, gratitude, and loving regard). In turn, this divide has led to a mind-body disconnection to food and eating that we believe is contributing to the pandemic of overeating and disordered eating.

In other words, Whole Person Integrative Eating is meant to be a bio-psycho-spiritual-social system that brings increasing awareness to the experience of food and eating, with a special focus on remedying the overeating styles.

The 7 Principles of Whole Person Integrative Eating

We designed the WPIE program so you can cultivate a dietary lifestyle comprised of the antidotes to the overeating styles: choosing fresh, whole food and eating it with positive emotions, mindfulness, gratitude, and loving regard in a pleasant social atmosphere, and with others. In other words, bringing self-awareness to food and eating makes it possible to have a Whole Person Integrative Eating practice that goes beyond the current what-and-how-much-to-eat model and instead expands the experience to include physical, emotional, spiritual, and social nourishment.

Here are the seven principles of our WPIE model and program:

1. *Positive feelings:* Release negative emotions before eating. Be aware of feelings before, during, and after eating.
2. *Appreciate food:* Have gratitude for food and its origins (such as the elements: water, earth, sunshine, etc.)—from the heart.
3. *Get fresh:* Eat fresh, whole food in its natural state as often as possible.
4. *Nourish your senses:* Focus on aroma, colors, flavors (sweet, sour, salty, etc.), texture, portion size, tactile sensations, even kinesthetic elements when you eat.
5. *Mindfulness eating:* Bring moment-to-moment, nonjudgmental awareness to every aspect of the meal.
6. *Amiable ambiance:* Eat in a positive psychological atmosphere and in pleasant aesthetic surroundings.
7. *Share fare:* Enjoy food-related experiences with others.

As you practice the seven principles of WPIE eating—and, more and more, you replace each of the seven overeating styles with the seven principles of Whole Person Integrative Eating—you create a dietary lifestyle that nourishes you multidimensionally. This section shows you how. As you look over the chart, keep in mind that an overeating style is simply a habitual pattern of eating—and that each overeating style is a continuum of eating behaviors that range from very poor to excellent. Scoring on the "poor" end means you're overeating a lot and are likely to gain weight, while scoring on the "excellent" end means less overeating and more normal weight.

Guide to the Overeating Styles versus Whole Person Integrative Eating

To get you started in the Whole Person Integrative Eating dietary lifestyle we tell you about in this section of the book, below is an infographic that puts it all together. The chart shows you the practice of

Whole Person Integrative Eating as opposed to the elements of the new-normal overeating styles we've identified. The goal is to replace an overeating-style relationship with food with the Whole Person Integrative Eating practice I tell you about throughout this section of the book.

To learn and understand the members of the overeating styles family versus the members of the Whole Person Integrative Eating dietary lifestyle, look over the chart below. It includes the overeating styles and the seven principles of our WPIE model and program as the remedies ("Overeating Styles Rx") for each overeating style. I organized the infographic based on the strongest to the least strong overeating styles.

Overeating Styles
versus
Whole Person Integrative Eating

The OVEREATING STYLES	Core Principles: WHOLE PERSON INTEGRATIVE EATING
#1. Overeating Style **Emotional Eating** Turning to food to manage negative feelings, such as anxiety and depression.	**#1. Emotional Eating Rx** **Positive Feelings** Be aware of feelings and thoughts before, during, and after eating.
#2. Overeating Style **Food Fretting** Dieting. Judging food as "good" or "bad." Over-concern about the "best" way to eat.	**#2. Food Fretting Rx** **Appreciate Food** Appreciate food and its origins — from the heart.
#3. Overeating Style **Fast Foodism** A diet of mostly fast, processed, fried, high-calorie foods.	**#3. Fast Foodism Rx** **Get Fresh** Eat fresh, whole food in its natural state as often as possible.
#4. Overeating Style **Sensory Disregard** Not savoring scent, flavor, colors, etc., or "flavoring" food with loving regard.	**#4. Sensory Disregard Rx** **Savor and "Flavor" Food** **with Loving Regard** Savor flavors, aromas, colors, and the mystery of life in food when you eat.

**#5. Overeating Style
Task Snacking**
Eating while doing other activities: working, driving, watching TV, etc.

**#5. Task Snacking Rx
Mindfulness Eating**
Bring moment-to-moment, nonjudgmental awareness to every aspect of the meal.

**#6. Overeating Style
Unappetizing Atmosphere**
Eating in unpleasant psychological and aesthetic surroundings.

**#6. Unappetizing Atmosphere Rx
Amiable Ambiance**
Eat in pleasant psychological and aesthetic surroundings.

**#7. Overeating Style
Solo Dining**
Dining alone most of the time.

**#7. Solo Dining Rx
Share Fare**
Enjoy food experiences with others.

Familiarize yourself with core components of the overeating styles and WPIE by comparing the major differences between the two styles of eating. The takeaway: this infographic is a guide for replacing the new normal food choices and eating behaviors that lead to overeating, overweight, and obesity with the elements of Whole Person Integrative Eating. As you practice the elements of WPIE we tell you about in this section, you create an enjoyable and nourishing experience each time you eat.

Putting Whole Person Integrative Eating into Action

What we are suggesting with the Whole Person Integrative Eating dietary lifestyle is this: we believe that our Whole Person Integrative Eating program is a paradigm-shifting, re-visioning of nutritional health that takes you beyond the purely physical and biological side of nutrition, weight loss, and well-being, to include the psychological, spiritual, and social whole-person ingredients so vital to health and healing.

In chapters 6–13, you'll also discover how to integrate each element of the WPIE dietary lifestyle into each eating experience. We suggest you consider making good friends with members of the WPIE family, because they empower you to take proactive steps to halt and reverse the relatively recent cultural shift of time-saving, eating-on-the-run, chemical-laden cuisine—trends and members of the overeating-styles family that are unequivocally contributing to our growing girth.

But perhaps even more important to your health and healing is this: As you practice integrating each element of the Whole Person Integrative Eating dietary lifestyle into your everyday eating experience, it is our hope you are inspired to re-envision your relationship to food, eating, and weight . . . so that each time you eat, you are nourished . . . for life.

CHAPTER 6

EMOTIONAL EATING Rx: POSITIVE FEELINGS

EMOTIONAL EATING Rx

Positive Feelings

Whole Person Integrative Eating
Practice #1

Be aware of feelings and thoughts before, during, and after eating.

Jessica was at work when she was blind-sided by her most recent emotional-eating episode. Nothing specific had happened to set it off. She was putting the final touches on her latest project report, when—WHAM!—she was overwhelmed by anxiety. What would happen if her report wasn't good? Would she miss out on a possible promotion? Would her colleagues lose respect for her? Would she be fired? Her carb-craving hit—hard.

Jessica had been on a diet and had been "good" for a week (see chapter 7 for more about overcoming dieting and the "Food Fretting" overeating style). Now she was about to blow it. On autopilot, without a second thought, she walked out of the high-rise office building and headed straight to her favorite deli. Five chocolate-chip cookies would do it. After wolfing them down in the privacy of her car in the parking lot, she felt calmer; the anxiety had diminished. Jessica returned to her office and to her nearly finished report.

Anne, too, is an emotional eater, but her overeating experience is much different from Jessica's. Anne's nighttime binge eating typically starts after work with a trip to the supermarket to buy bags of potato chips, a couple of pints of ice cream, and chunks of her favorite chocolate. Then she heads home, changes into comfortable clothes, and turns on the TV. Settling into bed surrounded by her favorite foods, she begins what she describes as "zoning out"—eating until she feels calmer—often to the point of falling in and out of sleep well before bedtime.

Although this is a typical evening for Anne, three hours after starting her binge she is amazed to find that she has finished all the food (products). On a not-quite-conscious level, she senses the chips and chocolate allay her anxiety in some way. She's also concerned about these binges because she wants to lose fifty pounds and stop zoning out, but she hasn't figured out how to accomplish this. Dieting hasn't helped, nor have willpower or the techniques she's read about in self-help books. In the meantime, Anne remains frustrated about her weight and is vaguely depressed and distressed and dependent on food binges to manage her darker moods.

Both Jessica and Anne are emotional eaters. Each turns to high-carb comfort foods to soothe negative emotions.

Emotional Eating: A "Family" of Negative Feelings

Most of us are familiar with the phrase "emotional eating," turning to comfort food to soothe negative feelings such as depression, anxiety, or anger, but also sometimes to enhance joyous, celebratory feelings in response, let's say, to a birthday or promotion. If you often experience out-of-control eating to manage your feelings and to self-soothe—in other words, for reasons other than having a healthy appetite—it's likely you're an emotional eater.[1]

If you are, this matters a lot to you and your weight, because out of the seven overeating styles Larry and I identified, Emotional Eating surfaced as *the* strongest predictor of overeating—*and* the number-one contributor of weight gain. Indeed, although all seven overeating styles are significantly linked to overeating and becoming overweight and obese, Emotional Eating was leaps and bounds ahead of the others as a predictor for overeating and weight gain.

Another powerful insight is this: Emotional Eating is just a nose length ahead of the Fast Foodism overeating style in predicting obesity. Put another way, the two overeating styles of Emotional Eating and Fast Foodism are the strongest drivers of overeating and becoming overweight and obese.[2]

Shedding still more light on this overeating style is the family of negative emotions we identified[2-4] that are strongly linked with the likelihood of an emotional-eating episode. Here they are, ranked from highest to lowest: anxiety, frustration, depression, sadness, and anger. And though it's not exactly an emotion, we define "food cravings" as the sixth negative emotion in the Emotional Eating overeating style.[3] Think of these negative emotions like genes shared by close siblings. If you experience one emotion, such as depression, you are also more likely to experience other emotions such as frustration, anxiety, or anger.

The WPIE Training Effect on Emotional Eating

With yet another twist of our statistical kaleidoscope, we gleaned insights into *improvements* emotional eaters made—in both overeating and weight loss—after they completed my six-week, eighteen-lesson e-course on Whole Person Integrative Eating.[5,6] Our key finding: the combination of reducing negative feelings and improving food choices were the strongest predictors of how much weight people lost. In other words, feelings and food choices are key factors in controlling weight.

Overeating. Emotional eaters trained in the Whole Person Integrative Eating dietary lifestyle substantially reduced their overeating episodes in response to one or more of the five negative feelings we identified. In other words, they were less inclined to be driven to overeat when a negative emotion hit. We also discovered that those who experienced fewer emotional-eating episodes also switched from eating a lot of processed, fried, and sweet foods when driven to overeat, to eating more vegetables and legumes.[7]

Overweight and obesity. The combination of reducing overeating episodes in response to negative feelings *and* eating fewer processed, fried, sweet foods and more plant-based foods was strongly linked with how much weight emotional eaters lost. [7]

In other words, we discovered this powerful combination: Emotional Eaters trained in the Whole Person Integrative Eating program 1) reduced their overeating episodes in response to negative emotions, 2) and they replaced high-carb, high-sugar, processed foods with smarter food choices that included more veggies and legumes. The end result: participants in the study experienced less overeating and more weight loss. [7]

Such findings about the Emotional Eating overeating style from our online WPIE course replicate a study we told you about in chapter 1. Recall that seventy-five health-psychology students at San Francisco State University completed the overeating style profile both prior to and after the two one-hour lectures I gave about Whole Person Integrative Eating. As with those who completed the online WPIE course, the students made significant reductions in each of the negative emotions that prompted them to overeat, they significantly *reduced* their frequency of eating fried foods and sweets, and they *increased* their intake of fruits and vegetables.[8] (See the appendix, "The Evolution and Science Behind the Overeating Styles," for more about the research on the overeating styles.)

We interpret these results to suggest that being exposed to the Whole Person Integrative Eating dietary lifestyle through two lectures, plus the "What's Your Overeating Style? Self-Assessment Quiz,"[9] was sufficient for students to significantly curtail their emotional-eating prompts, and to make smarter, healthier food choices.[8]

To up your odds of overcoming overeating driven by emotional-eating episodes, and to empower you to make deep, life-lasting changes in what and how you eat, this chapter gives you the latest Whole Person Integrative Eating research you can depend on to help turn Emotional Eating into a relationship to food, eating, and weight that nourishes the whole self each time you eat. We'll also give you scientifically sound insights into what influences negative emotions and in turn also influences emotional eating, plus evidence-based "transformation tips."

The key concept to keep in mind is this: the *antidote* to the Emotional Eating overeating style of the Whole Person Integrative Eating dietary lifestyle we tell you about in this chapter is designed to work *synergistically* with *all* elements of the Whole Person Integrative Eating lifestyle. These are the *what* you eat (food choices) and *how* you eat (eating behaviors) ingredients of the Whole Person Integrative Eating dietary lifestyle.

We begin the story about overcoming Emotional Eating with a WPIE study done with people with type 2 diabetes. When research participants replaced *all* the overeating styles—especially Emotional

Eating—with the other *how* components (eating behaviors) of Whole Person Integrative Eating, they received unexpected health benefits.

Derailing Diabetes with the "Family" of WPIE Eating Behaviors

Is it possible that replacing the overeating style of Emotional Eating with the *how*-you-eat elements of Whole Person Integrative Eating (positive feelings, mindfulness, gratitude, loving regard, and social connection)—influences not only what you eat, how much you eat, and what you weigh but also blood-sugar levels (HbA1c)? This is the question diabetes researchers Erica Oberg and Ryan Bradley posed when they applied the overeating styles and the WPIE dietary lifestyle to people with type 2 diabetes.

You may recall their research, which we told you about in chapter 1, when Oberg taught ten people with type 2 diabetes the Whole Person Integrative Eating program,[10] which included their taking our "What's Your Overeating Style? Self-Assessment Quiz."[9] What Oberg and Bradley found was this: they made the unusual and unexpected discovery that improvements in Emotional Eating *and* in the other behavioral *how*-you-eat overeating styles of WPIE (Food Fretting, Fast Foodism, Sensory Disregard, Task Snacking, Unappetizing Atmosphere, and Solo Dining) were stronger indicators of lower blood-sugar levels than *what* study participants ate![11,12]

At the start of the study, those with high Emotional Eating scores (Emotional Eating was a big issue for many in the study) had the higher baseline blood-sugar levels. But as participants made improvements in all the overeating styles, and in Emotional Eating especially—plus in their total overeating style score—blood-sugar levels decreased. Surprisingly and unexpectedly, macronutrient content—such as carbohydrate, protein, and fat intake—had a lesser influence on blood-sugar levels than improving overeating-style *behaviors* (such as Emotional Eating, Sensory Disregard, and Unappetizing Atmosphere).

Says lead investigator Oberg: "We taught the research participants about the seven overeating styles and those that made the biggest changes in their eating behaviors had the biggest improvements in blood sugar, independent of calories or carbohydrate intake. Literally, *how* [italics mine] they ate mattered more than *what* [italics mine] they ate," says Oberg.[13]

Such groundbreaking findings suggest that overcoming negative feelings linked with Emotional Eating[2]—as well as the other overeating styles—may be even more important determinants of how food is metabolized and of health and well-being than what you eat! In other words, Oberg's pioneering finding is that the *how* elements of WPIE (eating with others in a pleasant psychological and aesthetic atmosphere, with positive emotions, mindfulness, appreciation, and loving regard) were more significant predictors of lower blood-sugar levels than *what* research participants with type 2 diabetes ate.[11,12]

HALT: Overeaters Anonymous Meets Emotional Eating

You may be surprised that the term "emotional eating" didn't exist in the culture as recently as fifty years ago. If you often overate or binged to cope with unpleasant emotions—or because you were undereating or dieting to the point of being ravenous[6]—there was nowhere to turn for help. Although the term wasn't in the culture in 1960 when Overeaters Anonymous (OA) was founded, the concept was. "HALT" was already in use by Alcoholics Anonymous and was borrowed by OA. An organization that offered a twelve-step recovery program for compulsive overeating and other eating disorders, OA warned its members against becoming too Hungry, too Angry, too Lonely, or too Tired—because when you're feeling HALT emotions and you're an overeater, such emotions may trigger a binge.

OA understood that feeling HALT meant you are more likely to seek relief by overeating high-carb, sugary foods: if you become too hungry, too many cookies may override healthful food choices, chips may suppress anger, ice cream may soothe loneliness, or you may befriend french fries when you feel tired. Whatever the emotional upset, in place of giving yourself what you really need, you choose food and compulsive overeating as your solution.[14]

OA was way ahead of its time when, in the 1960s, it linked negative HALT emotions with the tendency of overeaters to turn to food for comfort. Today, "emotional eating" is a mainstream term used by many to describe the drive behind eating to cope and to feel better when unpleasant emotions such as depression and anxiety emerge.

Today, some health professionals describe the Emotional Eating overeating style as "compulsive overeating," "food addiction," or "self-medicating." No matter what it's called, many of us turn to food to relieve unpleasant, unwelcome emotions. Why? Because it works.

The Food-Mood Connection

The idea that the food you eat can actually soothe your mood—that the emotions you're experiencing may motivate you to make certain food choices—was given the scientific stamp of approval in the 1970s when Judith Wurtman, Ph.D., a scientist at the Massachusetts Institute of Technology (MIT), uncovered a fascinating facet of the emotional-eating enigma. Call it "nutritional neuroscience," "psychoneuro-immunology," "the study of food and mood," or "Psychological Nutrition"—my term for it, one of the "four facets of food" discussed in the introduction—Wurtman launched a new field of nutritional research that has confirmed what many of us know intuitively: what you eat affects your mind and mood, your tendency to pile on pounds, even your quality of life.

When Wurtman and her husband, Richard Wurtman, M.D., also a researcher at MIT, first linked food with mood, it was based on their discovery that both naturally occurring sugar and starch in carbohydrate foods (such as potatoes) as well as sugar added to food products (such as cookies and cake) elevate a powerful, naturally occurring chemical in your brain called serotonin.[15]

Even more fascinating was their discovery about the impact serotonin and other neurotransmitters (substances that pass information from cell to cell in the brain) have on your every mood, emotion, and food craving. For instance, about twenty minutes after you eat a carbohydrate-rich food, your brain releases serotonin; in turn, you feel more relaxed and calm. Want to feel more perky? Consume a lean, high-protein food such as fish, and the substance that's released (norepinephrine) lets you feel more awake and energetic (unlike the kick you get from caffeine, you're not stimulated, just more alert).

The Food-Mood Syndrome: It's a Vicious Cycle

Here is where the food-mood link to Emotional Eating really gets interesting. Since the Wurtmans' research, many studies have provided strong clinical evidence that carbohydrates can be calming, that protein-based foods can perk you up, and that certain fats in food end up as endorphins—substances in the brain that produce pleasurable feelings.

But there's another side to food-mood research. Yes, we now know that high-carb foods such as cookies and cake release serotonin, which can calm and relax you (this is likely why you choose the carrot cake instead of the carrot). But we also know that the sugary and sweet or crunchy and fried processed food products that emotional eaters most often choose to get a serotonin high actually contribute to deficiencies in certain vitamins and minerals that can cause your emotions to plummet, leading to a serious case of the doldrums.[16]

In this way, the food-mood syndrome that emotional eaters experience can become a vicious emotional cycle. You're feeling down, so you reach for, say, a prepackaged brownie. Sure, the brownie's sugar and white flour will soothe and calm you, but its high sugar content has a hidden side effect: it can actually deplete some nutrients that could help combat depression. In other words, the sweet concoction may somehow soothe your soul momentarily, but isn't it ironic that at the same time, it may also contribute to anxiety, depression, and other unpleasant emotions?

Chocolate: Elixir of Love . . . and Weight Loss?

No discussion about Emotional Eating, food, mood, and weight would be complete without pausing to savor the emotional ambrosia associated with choice chocolate. As science continues to focus its microscope on chocolate, especially dark chocolate with a high cocoa content, we're discovering its many delights: positive feelings, enhanced heart health, and most recently, increased odds of staying slim.

A natural high. Anyone who has experienced the emotional ambrosia associated with choice chocolate knows it lives up to its reputation as an aphrodisiac. Here's why. When you consume the sweet-and-creamy concoction of cocoa—the main ingredient in chocolate—combined with sugar and fat, blues-busting endorphins—naturally occurring substances (hormones) that function as painkillers and produce pleasurable feelings —are released in the brain, as is soothing serotonin.

Such mood enhancers are compounded by the phenylethylamine (PEA) in chocolate, a substance that likely enhances the release of endorphins. Indeed, the PEA released when you eat chocolate is the same PEA that produces its euphoric side effects when you fall in love.

Heart-healthy benefits. Apparently dark chocolate's high levels of cocoa flavonoids—antioxidants that mop up artery-clogging chemicals in the body—may help reduce heart disease by protecting blood vessels from damaging substances called free radicals. And other antioxidants in chocolate, called polyphenols, lower cholesterol, blood-sugar levels, and blood pressure, linking it with a lower risk of dying from a heart attack.

Less weight gain. Can the benefits of chocolate get even better? It seems so. When researchers surveyed one thousand adults with an average age of fifty-seven, they discovered that those who exercised regularly (an average of 3.6 times a week) and ate chocolate regularly (5 times a week) had a lower body mass index (BMI)—one BMI point lower, which is roughly five to seven pounds—than those who ate chocolate less often. And chocolate eaters weighed less even though they consumed more total calories and more saturated fat than less frequent chocolate eaters.

What might be the reason for this metabolic mystery? The secret "slimming ingredient" in chocolate that amps up metabolism is the antioxidant epicatechin. And this antioxidant powerhouse seems to work its weight-loss wonders by boosting energy-producing elements of the body's cells.

Reaping the rewards depends on choosing the right kind and the right amount of chocolate.

Right kind. Dark chocolate, dark chocolate, dark chocolate. And the darker the better, meaning you should choose chocolate with a cocoa content that's 70 percent or higher.

Right amount. You only need a small amount of dark chocolate to access its stay-slim effects. Choose about an ounce of dark chocolate each day, about the size of a credit card. Instead of measuring, try this simple guideline: If the piece of chocolate is thick, have one piece; if it's thinner and smaller, enjoy two or three pieces.

Ancient Food Wisdom Meets Modern Microbiome Science

So far in this chapter, I've told you about 1) the link Overeaters Anonymous made in the 1960s between negative emotions and overeating (its HALT model); 2) researcher Judith Wurtman's discovery in the 1970s about the food-mood connection; 3) and more recent research about the up-then-down influence of specific substances in food that influence both positive and negative emotions.

Now we're fast-forwarding to the twenty-first century, to a life-changing, groundbreaking, national research project that has given us pioneering, quantum-leap, newly discovered insights into what may be the *underlying causes* of many negative emotions, such as anxiety, depression, and food cravings (which, based on our research, we've defined as a negative feeling) that often lead to Emotional Eating episodes.

But first—to give you context about these pioneering research findings—a brief digression:

In the introduction, I told you about the discovery of Whole Person Integrative Eating. In the chapter, I mentioned that prior to the evolution of nutritional science in the early 1900s, ancient food wisdom from the world religions, cultural traditions, and Eastern healing systems—traditional Chinese medicine (TCM), India's Ayurvedic medicine, and Tibetan medicine—provided optimal-eating guidelines to humankind for millennia.

I am reminding you about this ancient food wisdom now because I want to bring your attention to this key concept: for thousands of years, the core belief of these Eastern medical systems has been that health—of both mind and body—begins with a healthy gut. As a matter of fact, more than 2,500 years ago, Greek physician Hippocrates—often called the "father of Western medicine"—said that all disease begins in the gut.

Today, modern nutritional science is verifying that the health of your gut and the foods you eat or don't eat have a profound effect on all aspects of your health, including your emotions, especially anxiety and depression, the two key negative feelings linked with Emotional Eating.

The science that is verifying the profound influence of gut health on your mind-body health evolved from the Human Microbiome Project (HMP).[17] Launched in 2007, the ten-year project received $170 million in funding from the National Institutes of Health Common Fund. Its purpose was twofold: to identify and define the human microbial flora, then to illuminate its role in health and disease.

What exactly is the microbiome, and why is it pivotal to your emotional health? In chapter 8, "Fast Foodism Rx: Get Fresh," I tell you about the influence of your microbiome and gut bacteria on weight and physical health.

Here, let's uncover the science that is now verifying what our ancient-food ancestors discovered centuries ago about the pivotal role your gut also plays in your emotional well-being.

Lifestyle, Emotions, and the Microbiome

Here are some gut-mood insights we didn't know until this century:

- Certain bacteria in your gut can help against depression and anxiety.
- Gut microbiota for people with depressive disorders is different from normal people.
- Some gut bacteria help produce chemicals called neurotransmitters, chemical messengers that help regulate our moods. Research is rapidly emerging about the gut microbiome—home to over thirty-five thousand bacterial species living in our digestive system that have a huge impact *on our emotions.*

Have you ever been so anxious about something, say, a presentation or final exam, that you lost your appetite? If so, you've experienced the "microbiome-gut-brain connection," the impact your thoughts and feelings have on your gut and the *microbiome* (*micro* means "small"; *biome* means "a habitat of living things") that is at the center of your gut. Because of recent research on the microbiome, we also know the gut-mood link is a two-way street: not only do your thoughts and feelings influence the gut bacteria in your gut, your gut bacteria can also modulate your emotions. How amazing! Today, science is verifying what Hippocrates and Eastern healing systems discovered centuries ago.

Our gut microbiome is made up of ten to one hundred trillion bacteria, fungi, and viruses: a complex ecosystem of microorganisms that live in our digestive systems. And these trillions of organisms play a powerful role in up to 90 percent of your physical and mental health. Throughout your life, the daily lifestyle you live (diet, stress, physical activity, social support, sleep, etc.) influences your microbiome and in turn your health.

This is because the foods you eat, your stress levels, toxins in your everyday environment, physical activity, social connection, and the quality of your sleep all work together to create variations and changes in the composition of your gut microbiota. These lifestyle influences can either keep you emotionally or physically healthy or, conversely, contribute to a plethora of mind-body diseases—from anxiety, depression, obesity, and cancer to arthritis and more. The determinant? The balance of "good" and "bad" microbes in your microbiome.

The "Good," the "Bad," and the Microbiome

Frontier research on the microbiome is revealing that the gut micro-biota does even more than influence weight (which we tell you about in chapter 7) and physical health: it also has a strong impact on brain health and in turn mood disorders such as anxiety and depression—the negative emotions that often lead to an Emotional Eating episode. Indeed, state-of-the-art research is revealing that negative emotions may drive you to eat because of the effect the gut microbiome has on the central nervous system, which communicates with the brain to regulate behavior.[18] Here's how it works.

Your gut microbiota influences the way your brain functions by communicating with your nervous system through *neurotransmitters*, naturally occurring chemical messengers that transmit signals throughout your mind-body. Poor gut health, meaning too much "bad" bacteria—or, put another way, a decrease in "good" gastro-intestinal bacteria—sends messages to your brain that could lead to mood and stress-related disorders, such as anxiety and depression.[19,20] In addition to mood disorders, a proliferation of bad bacteria also increases odds of inflammation and dozens of physical conditions—from stress-related irritable bowel syndrome and inflammatory bowel disease to cognitive decline (Alzheimer's), autoimmune diseases (arthritis), cancer, and more.[21]

Conversely, "good" gut-friendly bacteria can help to manage gut-brain communication in a positive way, meaning that an adequate balance of good gut bacteria can function as natural antidepressants and anti-anxiety organisms. Earlier in the chapter, we told you about food-mood research that links naturally occurring neurotransmitters, released throughout your body when you eat, that help regulate mood. Serotonin, one such neurotransmitter, is an antidepressant neurotransmitter, and about 80 percent of serotonin is produced in the gut.

This tells us that if your microbiome has a balance (homeostasis) of bacteria, emotions too are likely balanced, making you less prone to depression[22] and making it easier for you to handle stressful situations and negative emotions. If the food you eat is nutrient dense and whole (as are fresh, whole fruits, veggies, whole grains, legumes, nuts and seeds, and grass-fed, free-range animal-based foods), it is likely to have a beneficial effect on your microbiome and in turn your emotions; conversely, nutrient-deficient foods (processed, fried, high sugar, etc.) are likely to influence your microbiome and emotions negatively.

SAD and the Mind-Microbiome Cycle

What do industrial farming, farmed fish, pesticides, herbicides, additives, preservatives, and denatured, processed, junk, and fast food with low nutrient availability and lots of added chemicals have in common? They are all part of Western dietary changes over the last seventy years that threaten the stability of both your emotions and your microbiome. What I mean is this: by contributing to the excess of bad bacteria in your microbiome, today's standard American diet has a negative impact on your gut health, which in turn can contribute to mood problems like depression and anxiety. But negative emotions alone can also damage gut microflora and create an excess of "bad" microbes. The end result: the mind-microbiome cycle continues.

In other words, if you turn to fast, sugary, processed food to cope with unpleasant feelings—which, as mentioned earlier in this chapter in the "Food-Mood" section, can be calming—you're also feeding the bad bacteria in your gut (which loves sugar) and the odds of igniting more negative emotions. So yes, processed carbs may be soothing, but they can also create imbalances in your gut microbiota that can make you even more prone to anxiety and depression and ensuing Emotional Eating episodes.

The good news is that you have a lot of control over the health and balance of your microbiome and in turn your emotions, because the food you choose has a lot to do with the balance of both your microbiome and your emotions. The following "transformation tips" guide you to the foods that can help you overcome negative feelings—and to other Whole Person Integrative Eating strategies that lower your odds of Emotional Eating episodes while increasing your odds of overcoming overeating, overweight, and obesity.

6 Transformation Tips to Overcome Emotional Eating

Right now, you may be at a turning point as you read this section on strategies to overcome the Emotional Eating overeating style. You may embrace the idea of change and transformation in your relationship to food. Or resist it because you fear losing a valuable "friend" (food) or because you believe you may find it too much of a challenge to make the transformation to the dietary lifestyle we're telling you about in this book.

We understand: change isn't easy. We also understand the following:

- Those in our study who practiced our Whole Person Integrative Eating program turned to food less often when they experienced negative emotions. They also chose fresh food more frequently over fried and sugar-laden foods, and they lost weight.[2]
- Health-psychology students at San Francisco State University who learned the WPIE program via two lectures and filling out the "What's Your Overeating Style? Self-Assessment Quiz" (chapter 3) made significant reductions in each of the negative emotions that prompted them to overeat. They too reduced their frequency of eating fried foods and sweets and increased their intake of fruits and vegetables.[8]
- People with type 2 diabetes who made improvements in the behavioral overeating styles—in Emotional Eating especially—improved their total overeating style score and lowered their blood-sugar levels. Improving how they ate had a stronger influence on blood-sugar levels than what they ate.[11,12]

These studies remind us that Emotional Eating is one of seven members of the overeating styles "family" that has reshaped our cultural food landscape (well, food *product* landscape, actually), our waistlines, and our health in very unwelcomed ways. The antidote? Find a new family, one with Whole Person Integrative Eating members who have your best mind-body health interests . . . and waistline . . . at heart.

To begin: Familiarize yourself with the "transformation tips" that follow. Let these suggestions give you the insights and support you need to move past emotional struggles that are "in your head," so that instead you are discovering how to eat *from* your heart.

Remember, these and all the other WPIE guidelines in Part Two of this book are a lifetime practice. Think of the following transformation tips as the start of your WPIE journey toward well-being that can help you overcome the urge to splurge over time—they're not a quick-fix. Be patient with yourself. Be kind. Be compassionate. Self-growth can be one of life's most challenging . . . and fulfilling journeys.

1. Emotional Eating Rx: Positive Feelings

I started this chapter by highlighting the WPIE Emotional Eating guideline: *be aware of feelings and thoughts before, during, and after eating*. Not only is this the perennial Psychological Nutrition principle of WPIE, it's a strong first step toward overcoming Emotional Eating. Why? How might tuning into your feelings and thoughts not only before bingeing, but also during and after, help with Emotional Eating?

The first benefit: by identifying your feelings *before* giving into a food craving, you're taking a moment to connect with the emotions that are driving you to dive into your favorite comfort food. And this can also be an opportunity to check into what you "feel" like eating to fine-tune your moods and emotions.

What's the reason for checking into your feelings *during* an Emotional Eating episode? Earlier in this chapter I told you about the food-mood connection: the discovery in the 1970s that certain nutrients, such as carbohydrates, release chemical messengers that can calm and relax you (serotonin) or help you be more alert (dopamine). But here's the caveat: it takes about twenty minutes for your mind-body to register the soothing serotonin effects of say, the high-carb, sugary cookie you just ate; or the perk-you-up benefits of dopamine, which can be released when you eat, say chocolate. (Please see the sidebar, "Chocolate: Elixir of Love," for more about the many sensory and psychological delights of chocolate.)

After the food-mood effect has kicked in, why not take the time to enjoy, savor, and delight in the calm, pleasant feelings you're experiencing? In this way, you're both accessing and filling yourself with positive emotions, and making a mind-body, feel-good connection to food and the experience of eating.

2. Be B-Wise

While most of us try to cope with our negative emotions, food, and weight with the Emotional Eating overeating style, there are many other effective, proactive steps you can take. For instance, consider becoming B-wise. From dreary doldrums to a deeper depression, various B vitamins (there are eight)—including B1, B2, niacin, folate, and B12—can help you bust the blues. As a step toward defeating depression, consider the following B-wise guidelines when deciding which foods to eat.

Choose fresh, whole foods. A deficiency in one of the B vitamins, folate in particular, is linked to depression, as are other B-family relatives that are processed out of refined foods: B6, niacin, and B12. Some especially good B-abundant blues busters are unprocessed, unrefined grains (oats, millet, brown rice, etc.), fruits, vegetables, beans, nuts, and seeds. Vitamin B-rich greens such as spinach are especially good for this. (See "Mind Your Microbiome," below, and chapter 8, "Fast Foodism Rx: Get Fresh," for more about the mind-body benefits of fresh, whole foods.)

Shake the sugar habit. Consuming a lot of refined white sugar both damages and destroys B vitamins in the body; in this way, it contributes to deficiencies. Eliminate sugar from the diet, and depression often lifts—although why this is so isn't well understood. One theory is that the "high" a person derives from sugar is due to elevated glucose (blood sugar) and endorphins, which produce feelings of relaxation and euphoria. When a diet is rich in foods loaded with the B vitamins and low in sugar, the levels of B vitamins, glucose, and endorphins remain stable, reducing the chances of depression (see "Mind Your Microbiome," below, for more about high-sugar foods and mind-body health).

Avoid or limit alcohol or caffeine. Consuming too much alcohol and caffeine can cause the loss of certain B vitamins—and deficiencies of vitamins B6 and niacin especially can bring you down. Not only does excessive alcohol and caffeine consumption reduce the absorption of B vitamins, but too much of these beverages also contributes to protein and mineral deficiencies.

Many of us have felt sad or have had the Monday-morning blahs at times; others—more than sixteen million Americans[22]—experience serious depression during their lifetime. Include more foods high in the B vitamins (nuts and seeds, whole grains, dark, leafy vegetables), and you may improve your mood and be less likely to experience depression linked to Emotional Eating. (Please see chapter 8, "Fast Foodism Rx: Get Fresh," for more about this.)

3. Mind Your Microbiome

In "'The Good,' the 'Bad,' and the Microbiome" section above, I told you about the human microbiome and its far-reaching effects on emotions. Sometimes called your "second brain," the gut-brain connection is based on the trillions of cells that live inside your gut microbiota, which have the power to communicate directly with neurons in our brains.

The "good bacteria" in your gut keeps your immune system strong and protects you against a plethora of mind-body ailments.[23] But when microbiota is altered due to exposure to pollutants, toxins, high stress, and a poor diet, negative emotions such as depression and anxiety can be ignited. The solution? Gut-protective foods that are rich in anti-inflammatory antioxidants, minerals, and essential fatty acids—foods that can regulate and strengthen the microbiome and in turn your immune system.[24] In other words, when your gut is happy, you are happy. (For more insights about optimal eating, see chapter 8, "Fast Foodism Rx: Get Fresh.")

Here, gut-friendly foods to choose and gut-harming foods to avoid:

Choose gut-friendly foods. To ward off or even prevent negative emotions, choose chemical-free fresh foods that can feed good bacteria and keep them plentiful. A sampling:
- *Vegetables*—such as leafy greens, beets, celery, cauliflower, broccoli, brussels sprouts, onions, peas
- *Whole fruit*—such as red, blue, or black berries, cherries, pineapple, oranges, pears, strawberries, pomegranates
- *Ancient and whole grains*—such as amaranth, quinoa, buckwheat, millet, barley, oats
- *Beans/legumes*—black beans, chickpeas, lentils, Anasazi beans, adzuki beans, black-eyed peas
- *Nuts and seeds*—walnuts, chia seeds, flax seeds
- *Herbs, spices, tea*—turmeric, cayenne, ginger, cinnamon, cloves, rosemary, oregano, thyme, sage, green tea
- *Probiotic foods*—yogurt, kefir, kombucha, fermented vegetables
- *Animal foods*—wild fish (such as salmon and trout), grass-fed and free-range chicken, pasture-raised beef, cage-free eggs

Avoid gut-harming faux foods. For a happy gut and to enhance positive emotions, choose the fresh foods above as often as possible. Avoid fast, processed, refined, denatured, "chemical cuisine" foods. A sampling:

- *Fried foods*—french fries, potato chips, corn chips, chicken
- *Refined grains*—such as white-flour products, white rice, white corn
- *Processed oils*—that have been heated to high temperatures and that can sit on the grocery shelf for years
- *Sweets, sweets, sweets*—cookies, cake, donuts, soft drinks, colas
- *Packaged food products*—filled with more chemicals and ingredients you never heard of or can't pronounce when compared to fresh, whole, real foods that are microbiome-friendly

4. Quick-Fix Blues-Buster Recipes

Anxiety. Dieting. Bingeing on high-carb sweets. Millions of emotional eaters self-medicate their negative emotions such as depression and loneliness and their Food Fretting behaviors like dieting, obsessing about food and weight, and so on by overeating high-carb sweets that could actually calm unpleasant emotions, at least for the moment (see "The Food-Mood Connection" section above for more about this).

The good news is that there are other ways to cope with negative emotions that often lead to bingeing; there are ways to relate to them, contain them, and cope with them so that you are less and less driven to engage in self-medicating Emotional Eating. Meet the foods that may help. But first, a look at "downer" foods to avoid:

"Downer" foods. What are "downer" foods? In short, they are processed, fast, sugar- and fat-laden junk food—and they aren't really food; rather, they're food *products*. From cookies, cake, chips, and donuts to fries, ice cream, candy bars, and soda, comfort foods are often high in sugar, refined carbs (such as white flour), and mood- and health-harming fats. This means these often tasty, high-carb foods may provide some short-term comfort by releasing soothing serotonin, but you won't get long-term relief; rather, sugar-laden, denatured comfort food could worsen negative feelings because its high-sugar content can send your blood-sugar levels plummeting, leaving you even more depressed and fatigued than prior to eating them.

Damage control: carbs without the crash. Is it possible to consume high-carb, blues-busting foods that can calm you—even diminish depression—minus the "downer" aftermath? Absolutely. When you have the urge to splurge on sugary, processed, high-carb food products, choose *real food* to bust the blues. Here, some quick-fix blues busters:

Key Curb-the-Craving Concept

Be sure to wait at least twenty minutes after you eat to get the calming effects of serotonin. This is how long it takes for your brain to register that soothing serotonin is working its wonders.

- *Smoothie.* Combine two cups chopped dark leafy greens, one cup blueberries, three walnut halves, one cup milk of choice (such as dairy, almond, soy, etc.), half a cup juice of choice, one teaspoon flax oil. Blend.
- *Tapas.* Sauté minced garlic, chopped mushrooms, and chopped parsley, until soft. Spread some on toasted, crusty whole-grain bread.
- *Beans.* Roast already-cooked garbanzo beans and enjoy them as a snack. Or add them to a fresh green salad.
- *Bread.* Toast a piece of multigrain bread of choice. Sprinkle it with organic flax seed oil.
- *Cereal.* Enjoy a bowl of cracked oatmeal with a handful of blueberries and milk of choice.
- *Popcorn.* Air-pop some popcorn. Spritz lightly with water or olive oil. Sprinkle with a dash of salt and pepper. Toss.
- *Nuts/seeds.* Try a quarter cup of raw, unroasted nuts or seeds of choice. A sampling: walnuts, cashews, almonds, pumpkin or sunflower seeds.
- *Nut butter.* In a small saucer, add a tablespoon of raw, unroasted peanut, sesame (tahini), cashew, almond, or any other nut butter of choice. Drizzle a teaspoon of honey over the nut butter. Savor the flavors and creaminess.
- *Veggies.* Munch some carrots, celery, or cherry tomatoes; crunch Romaine lettuce leaves.
- *Dips and spreads.* Use the nut-butter blend above as a dip or spread for your veggies. Or try some hummus or guacamole as a dip.

5. WPIE: An Internal and External "Positive Emotion" Practice

"Be aware of feelings and thoughts before, during, and after eating" is the Whole Person Integrative Eating guideline for the Emotional Eating overeating style that starts this chapter. It's a simple yet revolutionary suggestion because it provides an opportunity for you to pause—even for a moment—before eating so you can check in with and be conscious of whatever negative feelings you're experiencing that may be leading you to an Emotional Eating episode.

This internal step of checking in with your feelings and thoughts before, during, and after eating may be the first step toward bringing positive feelings to the forefront of your relationship to food and eating. It is also the beginning of your discovery of the *internal* and *external* WPIE guidelines we tell you about throughout Part Two of this book, each of which can help you overcome all the overeating styles.[2,10]

Internal and External
WPIE PRINCIPLES

Internal WPIE Principles	*External* WPIE Principles
Positive feelings	Fresh whole food
Appreciation	Pleasing aesthetic environment
Mindfulness	Social connection
Loving regard	
Pleasant emotional atmosphere	

The powerful takeaway message in this chapter is that the elements of the Whole Person Integrative Eating practice address both the *internal* and *external* reasons you overeat. In other words, the food choices (*what* you eat) and eating behaviors (*how* you eat) of the entire WPIE dietary lifestyle show you how to replace negative emotions with more than positive feelings. They also guide you to nourish yourself with pleasure-filled food choices, thoughts, and eating behaviors each time you eat.

6. Meet the WPIE Guided Meal Meditation

I created the WPIE Guided Meal Meditation in chapter 13 to help you take charge of negative feelings each time you eat, so that more and more you can put into action the two key Whole Person Integrative Eating antidotes to Emotional Eating:

- Replace negative emotions with positive feelings when you eat.
- Be aware of your feelings and thoughts before, during, and after eating.

But the WPIE Guided Meal Meditation does more: along with helping you balance your emotions while eating, it also provides a guide to implementing all of the WPIE antidotes to the overeating styles.[25] In other words, the WPIE Guided Meal Meditation integrates both the internal and external elements of the Whole Person Integrative Eating dietary lifestyle, so you can practice the pleasures of Whole Person Integrative Eating each time you eat.

The next chapter, "Food Fretting Rx: Appreciate Food," gives you the insights you need to eat with gratitude—another internal ingredient of Whole Person Integrative Eating that helps you to cultivate the ability to eat for pleasure, with feel-good feelings and a healthy appetite—so you can overcome the Food Fretting overeating style and experience true nourishment each time you eat.

CHAPTER 7

FOOD FRETTING Rx: APPRECIATE FOOD

FOOD FRETTING Rx

Appreciate Food

Whole Person Integrative Eating
Practice #2

Be grateful for food and its origins—from the heart.

Gratitude is a gracious acknowledgment of all that sustains us,
a bow to our blessings, great and small.
Gratitude is not dependent on what you have.
It depends on your heart.[1]
—Jack Kornfield, "Gratitude and Wonder"

Are you a food fretter? Do you see yourself in any of the following examples of Food Fretting?

"I was good today," you may think when you've managed to avoid unhealthful foods, stick to your diet, under eat, or eat the "best" and healthiest food, or what you think you *should* eat.

"When my food cravings become powerful and I eat foods that are 'bad,' I feel so guilty" is typical self-think for many food fretters.

"She shouldn't eat that chocolate cake. Doesn't she have any willpower?" you might think as you watch someone eat what she 'shouldn't.'"

An obsession about food. Anxiety about the "best" way to eat. Counting calories. Dieting. Feeling gluttonous, bad, and guilty when you overeat. Food cravings. Judging others about their food choices. Feeling righteous when you eat what you think you *should*. The Food Fretting overeating style is a pattern of thoughts, feelings, and food-related actions that have one thing in common: obsessing about food and eating. These complex and dynamic elements of Food Fretting may be a key reason overeaters are often filled with mostly negative thoughts and feelings about food and eating.[2]

Yes, the Food Fretting overeating style—as with all the overeating styles we've identified—is linked with increased odds of overeating. But the mental and emotional stress and misery that obsessing about food causes by itself and its impact on the quality of your life may be reason enough to take the time to discover how to go from an in-your-head Food Fretting relationship to food and eating to instead the pleasure-filled, nourishing WPIE guideline to eat from your heart by being grateful for food and its origins. This chapter will show you how.

The WPIE Training Effect on Food Fretting

Those who took the online WPIE e-course[3] and completed the pre- and post-overeating styles questionnaire[4] made substantial improvements in their Food Fretting behaviors. This select group showed it is possible to reduce *all* ten elements of Food Fretting and in turn to reduce their overeating by learning and practicing the Whole Person Integrative Eating dietary lifestyle.[5]

Overeating. After participants filled out the "What's Your Over-eating Style? Self-Assessment Quiz,"[4] but prior to their taking the WPIE e-course, Larry and I looked at the Food Fretting elements that were most related with overeating frequency and weight gain. Five items stood out as particularly strong: anxiety about the "best" way to eat; food cravings; and feeling bad, guilty, or gluttonous in response to overeating.[6] After taking the e-course, those who reduced their over-eating were the ones who also reduced these three Food Fretting factors: food cravings, anxiety about the "best" way to eat, and obsession about food and eating.

Overweight and obesity. At the start of the WPIE e-course, the Food Fretting factors that were most related to being overweight and obese were food cravings, obsessing about food, and dieting. As with those whose overeating lessened, participants who lost weight after taking the online e-course over the six-week period reduced the three Food Fretting variables of food cravings, anxiety about the "best" way to eat, and obsessing about food.

The most telling insight from the Food Fretting overeating style is this: Those who completed the pre- and post-overeating styles quiz and the WPIE e-course reduced *all* ten elements of Food Fretting. In turn, they obsessed about food less and had fewer "side effects" of overeating, such as feeling stuffed; as a result, they lost weight. This makes sense based on our findings, because all ten Food Fretting items under the umbrella of obsessing about food are *intimately interrelated with one another*. For instance, if food fretters judge others about what they eat, they are also likely to feel bad when they themselves overeat, diet, have food cravings, and so on.[7] (See the appendix, "The Evolution and Science Behind the Overeating Styles," for more about the research on the overeating styles.)

The takeaway: the intricate network of food-fretting elements is strongly related to overeating. Therefore, by reducing even a few food-fretting factors, you are also likely to lessen other elements of the Food Fretting overeating style. In other words, lessening obsessive thoughts, feelings, and actions about food and eating helps lower your desire to overeat and increases your odds of weight loss.

Food Fretting: A New Normal Overeating Style

If you think the food fretter's relationship to food, eating, dieting, and weight loss is normal—you're right. In America, 75 percent of women have one or more of the ten elements of food fretters, meaning that they have obsessive thoughts, feelings, or behaviors related to food or their bodies;[8] 91 percent of college women have attempted to control their weight through dieting; 22 percent diet "often" or "always";[9] and half of nine to ten-year-old girls are dieting.[10]

The goal of food fretters, though, isn't always weight loss. Rather, many simply have a preoccupation about the "best" way to eat, to the point of obsession. Elements of this new-normal overeating style have become so common that the term *orthorexia* has been coined to describe it. The word comes from the Greek *orthos*, "correct or right," plus *orexis*, "appetite."

Although orthorexia hasn't been classified as an official eating disorder,[11] the National Eating Disorder Foundation says "orthorexics become fixated on food quality and purity. They become consumed with what and how much to eat, and how to deal with 'slip-ups' . . . they sometimes feel superior to others, especially in regard to food intake."[12]

The Food Fretting overeating style may include the concept of orthorexia, but it differs in that Food Fretting identifies a specific family of *obsessive* thoughts, feelings, and behaviors that are linked to increased odds of overeating, overweight, and obesity. These thoughts, feelings, and behaviors include counting calories; feeling anxiety about the "best" way to eat; having food cravings; feeling gluttonous, bad, and guilty when overeating; dieting; judging others about what and how they eat; obsessing about food; and feeling righteous when you eat what you *should*.

But there's the light at the end of the food-fretting tunnel: our research has revealed it's possible to reduce an obsession about food and your odds of overeating, overweight, and obesity by replacing an in-your-head, thought-filled relationship to food and eating with an appreciative, eating-from-your-heart, nourishing connection to food and to the extraordinary experience of eating.[13]

From "In Your Head" to Eating *"From* Your Heart"

Eating with mindfulness, gratitude, and loving regard are the three Spiritual Nutrition guidelines in the Whole Person Integrative Eating dietary lifestyle. Spiritual ingredient number two, the *appreciation* guideline, is the Whole Person Integrative Eating antidote to the Food Fretting overeating style that we're telling you about in this chapter.[13,14]

While eating with a sense of heartfelt gratitude may seem like an unusual remedy for overcoming the Food Fretting overeating style, consider life in the nineteenth century, when world religions guided people with a set of stable, time-honored, unquestioned, internalized religious and moral codes or ideals such as integrity, kindness, and compassion. Most people lived in small towns and rural communities then, where these values were reinforced by family, friends, faith, and community. With such internal values, many people said blessings of gratitude before eating.

By the twentieth century, life had changed. Today most of us live in or near urban centers, often far from our families, with little connection to our communities . . . or to where our food is grown. As science replaced religion as our higher "authority," success in life no longer means being guided by our internal values and the well-being of our community; rather, the criteria has shifted to external standards and a focus on the self, especially the image we present to the world: our accomplishments, our prestige, our clothes, our cars and homes—and our physical appearance. In the process, many of us have lost touch with our inner essence, our true selves.

Explains clinical psychologist Michael Mayer, Ph.D., "When we allow the craving for external images, such as being thin or looking perfect, to replace our more essential needs, such as our need for love, connectedness, learning, and right livelihood, then we become addicted to the sweets of life, rather than to the main meal, where true nourishment lies."[15] In other words, we miss out on the chance to foster true nourishment when we stop living from internal, heartfelt values; when we stop living *from* our heart and instead relate to life—including food and eating—from an external, in-your-head, Food Fretting perspective.

Eating From a "Place of Spirit"

In the West, many may describe the energy you experience when you're feeling internally nourished by gratitude as a release of endorphins, chemical "messengers" released in the brain that make us feel relaxed, connected, unanxious. In China, though, the concept of *chi*—the life force within all living things, from feelings to food—is used to describe such connection. Psychologist and Taoist meditation practitioner Michael Mayer calls it "the universal mother," that "energy potential in the world that is soothing, giving us a sense of merging with" the mysterious energy source that is life itself.[15] Indeed, the cultivation of chi is both an art and science, capable of unleashing insights, intuition, and a sense of unity—between mind, body, self, and the world.

We're suggesting that accessing chi through gratitude is a path to changing from a Food Fretting sensibility to a way of thinking about food and eating that nourishes you multidimensionally each time you eat. And it's possible to do this by accessing the Spiritual Nutrition antidotes inherent in Whole Person Integrative Eating: mindfulness, appreciation, and loving regard. In this chapter, we'll show you how to fill your thoughts *and heart* with gratitude and enjoyment of food, based on the original meaning of the word *diet*, which meant "way of life." In other words, integrate the Whole Person Integrative Eating practice of *gratitude* into your relationship with food and eating—from the heart—and you'll be taking yet another powerful step toward stopping overeating and creating a pleasurable, nourishing relationship to food and eating.

As you read this chapter, remember that the gratitude ingredient we're telling you about is one of seven WPIE guidelines that are based on an integration of ancient food wisdom and modern nutritional science. In this chapter, we'll introduce you to some of these ancient gratitude ingredients; research about their healing power and how they may help you overcome Food Fretting thoughts, feelings, and behaviors; and people who integrate an attitude of gratitude into their meals—and lives—every day.

The Ancient Power of Thankfulness

Yogi master Nischala Devi tells the story in the Hindu tradition that embodies the WPIE perennial principle of gratitude. It is a parable from India that suggests that an appreciative heart empowers food to open its treasures to you—to the degree that you are willing to open your heart to the silent message in your meals.

Once there was a great man, a saint, who had a devout wife. Early in their married life, she asked what she could do solely for him. He said, "The only thing I want you to do is this: every time you serve me a meal, also place a small bowl of water and a needle next to it." She honored his request over the fifty years of their marriage, though she never saw him use either the water or needle.

Toward the end of his life, he asked his wife if he had ever done anything to upset her, even a small thing. "I've been placing a small bowl of water and a needle next to your plate throughout our marriage," she said, "but I've never seen you use either. What's their purpose?"

He explained that he had such a deep appreciation for the food—and for the devotion with which she prepared it—he didn't want to waste a morsel. Should he drop even a single grain of rice on the table, he wanted to pick it up with the needle and wash it, so he could eat it and not waste it.[14]

Such deeply felt thankfulness for food (and all other gifts bestowed by the Creator of the universe) is also at the core of the cosmology of Native American nations. For instance, harvest festivals begin and end with prayers of thankfulness for all foods and other elements of nature. In this manner, forces such as scarcity and drought are believed to be diminished and replaced with abundant crops and other gifts of nature. Native Americans find themselves not only thankful for food; they're also grateful for the origins of food and the forces that create it: Creator or Great Spirit, and the spirit forces or elements of wind, thunder, lake, sun, moon, and the stars.

"Other-Oriented" Gratitude and Your Heart

The fact that heartfelt appreciation has been so integral to food and all aspects of life for thousands of years (as we've seen with Hinduism and Native American belief systems) isn't coincidental. "Gladdening the heart," often through appreciation, is an ancient, cross-cultural concept that has traveled throughout the ages in Egyptian scrolls and scripture, from the biblical Psalms to the Qur'an, Buddhism, and more. Gladdening the heart is believed to be balm for a troubled emotional heart—an antidote to negative emotions such as depression and anxiety (see chapter 6, "Emotional Eating Rx: Positive Feelings," for more about positive emotions).[16]

What makes thankfulness for our inter-beingness with food so powerful is the degree to which we may experience authentic, deep caring about food, from the heart. To care about food in such a way is inherently what co-author and behavioral scientist Larry Scherwitz, Ph.D., refers to as being "other-oriented." This means that instead of focusing on your own food-related concerns, you are paying attention to the food before you, regarding and appreciating the mystery of life it contains and provides. In other words, you're holding gratefulness in your heart for food and its origins rather than choosing foods solely because they're good for the heart (or waistline or mood and so on). When you do this, you're focusing on something other than yourself. And focusing on the "other," such as the food before you—instead of "self"—may actually help your heart health.

A startling new discovery by Larry reveals *self-involvement* is a major risk factor for heart disease; and conversely, an "other-oriented," appreciative worldview can lead to wellness.[17]

While many well-known lifestyle elements—such as diet, exercise, stress, and smoking—can contribute to heart disease, Larry has discovered a powerful new risk factor for heart disease he calls "self-involvement," measured by excessive use of the pronouns *I, me, my,* and *mine*. While taping the interviews of nearly six hundred men, a third of them with heart disease, Larry counted how often the men used first-person pronouns—*I, me, my, mine*. His breakthrough findings highlight self-involvement as a possible underpinning of heart disease, because self-involved people have a greater risk of dying when they have a heart attack.

With such findings, Larry challenges conventional thinking about the traditional risk factors for heart disease: not only is self-involvement a risk factor, *it was a stronger predictor of heart disease than most of the traditionally identified causes.* Apparently, self-involvement may increase the odds of an ongoing cascade of certain chemicals that profoundly affect heart health; indeed, they affect every system in the body, as well as our emotional, spiritual, and social well-being. These insights provide the key to understanding the health-*harming* effects of self-absorption and separation and, conversely, the health-*enhancing* phenomenon of other-awareness and the power to create connection through heartfelt gratitude.[17]

In other words, "other-oriented," appreciation-filled moments each time you eat—and throughout the day—may keep your heart healthy and balance emotions. Eating with a gladdening-the-heart consciousness may mean you are doing more than simply appreciating food; you are turning a self-involved, isolated self—a heart apart—into a self of healing connection. Intriguing research by the HeartMath Institute in Boulder Creek, California, supports this idea.

Heart Intelligence and Your Health

Since 1991, the opposite of a self-involved heart—an appreciative, loving heart—has been the focus of HeartMath. According to founder Doc Lew Childre and executive consultant Howard Martin: " . . . when heart intelligence (a term describing the concept that the heart is an intelligent system with the ability to balance our emotional and mental systems) is engaged [with positive emotions], it can lower blood pressure, improve nervous system and hormonal balance, and facilitate brain function."[18]

HeartMath researchers have also discovered that the heart's magnetic field (the *magnetic* influence of electrical currents and magnetized materials on nearby moving electrical charges) *radiates outside the body* and can affect other people.[19] This means that when your heart is filled with loving appreciation, those feelings affect your body's electromagnetic field, causing it to extend three or more feet from the body.[19] Such findings also bring up the possibility that this "heartfelt" electromagnetic field may somehow be infused into the meal before you.

What does this suggest about bringing an appreciative consciousness to meals? If you flavor your meals with other-oriented appreciation, spice them with heartfelt blessings, and infuse both yourself and the food with gratitude, you are choosing to "appreciate food and its origins—from the heart," over the in-your-head Food Fretting overeating style and its family members of dieting and obsessing about food and weight and the "best" way to eat.

In other words, when you cherish food and all aspects of the eating experience, you may also find that the healing, magical mystery of gratefulness will work through you, in you—and for your body, mind, and soul.

Appreciation Blessings

Over the centuries, heartfelt blessings, prayers, or simple moments of quiet contemplation have become humankind's ritualized ways of expressing gratitude for the life-sustaining nourishment food provides. These expressions of gratitude evolved as thanks not only for the measurable and visible but also for the invisible, immeasurable, alchemical, life-giving, and life-containing mystery inherent in food.

Opportunities to bless food can be found endlessly in everyday life. Whether you begin the day with a glass of orange juice, cup of coffee, or cereal; eat lasagna warmed by a microwave oven at work; snack on an apple; or eat light fare of steamed vegetables for dinner, each time you're around food, you have the opportunity to appreciate it. To begin, let go of worries, thoughts, plans, and so on (see chapter 6, "Emotional Eating Rx: Positive Feelings," for more about this). Then, inhaling deeply and exhaling slowly, invoke a feeling of heartfelt regard for your food and say a blessing.

A ZEN BLESSING FROM THICH NHAT HAHN

In this plate of food, I see the entire universe supporting my existence.

A JEWISH BLESSING OVER BREAD

Blessed art Thou, O Lord our God, Creator of the Universe, who brings forth bread from the earth.

FROM INDIA'S UPANISHADS

Let us be together; let us eat together. Let us be vital together; let us be radiating truth, radiating the light of life.

JAPANESE BLESSING

Before eating, say "itadakimasu" (I gratefully receive). *After finishing the meal, say* "gochisosama (deshita)" (thank you for the meal).

FROM SOUL FOOD RESTAURANTEUR PAMELA STROBEL

We are thankful for the triumph of soul food, "black folk cooking." Spiced with spirit and served from the heart, it transforms body and soul and helps spirit to soar.

EXCERPT FROM AN ISLAMIC PRAYER

Praise to Thee, Oh God, for allowing us to eat, drink and be satisfied with the food and the liquid.

INTEGRAL YOGA MEAL PRAYER

OM, Beloved Mother Nature,
You are here on the table as our food.
Endlessly bountiful;
Benefactress of all.
Please grant us health and strength,
Wisdom and dispassion to find
Permanent Peace and Joy, and to share that Peace and Joy with one and all.
Mother Nature is my mother
My Father is the Lord of All,
All creation is my family,
The entire universe is my home.
I offer this unto OM,
That Truth which is universal.
May the entire universe be filled with
Peace and Joy, Love and Light[20]

If you must eat quickly because of time constraints, consider shooting a prayer of gratitude at your food with the simple Native American Seneca greeting, "Thank you for being."

Attitudes of Gratitude: De-Food Fretting Strategies

There's a lot more you can do to "de-food fret" and overcome your food-related anxieties, self-recrimination, judgment, and guilt. Here are some suggestions to transcend the cycle of dieting and obsessing about food and weight.

Don't obsess about dieting. One consequence of ongoing dieting can be increased obsession about food, eating, and weight. Indeed, more and more research is linking traditional dieting with increased risk of weight gain. Consider *dieting* in the best sense of the word: as a way of life and eating we're telling you about in this book.

And consider this: from the perspective of the Whole Person Integrative Eating dietary lifestyle, food in itself is *not* "sinful," "good," "bad," "right," or "wrong"—unless you're projecting moral attributes onto it and onto yourself! Nor is food something to be counted, feared, and analyzed. In other words, I'm suggesting that, instead of viewing food through the lens of today's new normal of judgment, relate to it as an expression of the ancient meaning of the word *diet*, in the lens of Whole Person Integrative Eating: as a social, ceremonial, and sensual delight and as a gift that enhances your physical, emotional, spiritual, and social well-being each time you eat.

Stop counting calories compulsively. Traditional diets that ask you to restrict calories and to eat by the numbers (counting calories, fat grams, and so on) don't work for the long term. Counting calories by itself is not a problem; a compulsive and obsessive attitude about calories is. To lose weight, consider other ways of relating to food so that each time you eat you have an enjoyable experience that nourishes your entire being. Instead of staying lost in a maze of measurements, nutrients, and numbers, focus on fresh foods (see chapter 8, "Fast Foodism Rx: Get Fresh" for more about this), delicious flavors, the profound pleasure of eating, and the delight you take in dining with others. In other words, bring *heartfelt* appreciation to all aspects of the dining experience.

Give up guilt-tripping when you overeat. Guilt and its relatives—self-reproach, shame, remorse, and blame—are part of a food fretter's relationship to food. It's all about what is "right" and what is "wrong." Eat something "wrong" that isn't in your diet, that you "shouldn't" eat, or that tastes "sinful," and—if you're a food fretter—you're likely to respond with guilt.

Consider this: guilt isn't a real feeling. At its core lies the belief you've done something wrong, and now you must suffer for it. To break that conviction and get the upper hand over guilt, change what you choose to believe with the WPIE guideline of bringing heartfelt appreciation to food—and its origins. If you overeat, appreciate and savor the experience. Should you relapse, enjoy the experience—especially if it was with food you like! Finally, forgive yourself, for forgiveness is a necessity in any relationship—including the one you have with food. Then return to your usual Whole Person Integrative Eating dietary lifestyle.

Cease obsessing. If you're fixated on and preoccupied with food-related thoughts, feelings, and behaviors, if you think or worry about food or weight constantly and compulsively, you are obsessing. The way out is to step from the shade in which you're living, into the sunshine. Our WPIE Guided Meal Meditation in chapter 13 in this book can help you do this. It can show you how to replace obsessive, food-related thoughts and feelings with the nourishing guidelines (fresh food, positive feelings, mindfulness, gratitude, loving regard, and sharing) inherent in Whole Person Integrative Eating.

Cultivate awareness. To overcome Food Fretting, familiarize yourself with the strongest elements of food fretters: obsessing about food; anxiety about the "best" way to eat; food cravings; and feeling bad, guilty, or gluttonous in response to overeating. The second step: when one of these elements surfaces, cultivate awareness by having a self-monitoring strategy in place that you can turn to, such as keeping a log of any critical, judgmental, or obsessive thoughts you may have. Then pause, take a slow, deep breath, and let the thought pass on.

Heartfelt Attention

If you're often filled with obsessive, judgment-filled, Food Fretting thoughts about the "best" way to eat, dieting, calorie counting, and anxiety-related overeating, consider applying the stages-of-change concepts we told you about in chapter 4 to overcoming the Food Fretting overeating style. First, decide if you're really ready to change. If the answer is "yes," consider the pros and cons of your Food Fretting, then put a plan of action into place. Preparation before action is a key to success.

Ultimately, the key to successfully overcoming the Food Fretting overeating style is to create a positive, pleasure-filled relationship to food and eating by giving food nonjudgmental, heartfelt attention. Bringing an "appreciation consciousness" to the experience of food and eating and gladdening the heart with gratitude each time you eat can help you replace Food Fretting with the experience of actually enjoying food . . . and reducing your odds of overeating.

The next chapter, "Fast Foodism Rx: Get Fresh," is the third ingredient, the next practice in our Whole Person Integrative Eating dietary lifestyle. In it, you will discover state-of-the-art insights into foods that contribute to overeating—and why they do—and the food choices that can lead naturally to weight loss, health, and healing—and why.

CHAPTER 8

FAST FOODISM Rx: GET FRESH

FAST FOODISM Rx

Get Fresh

Whole Person Integrative Eating
Practice #3

Eat fresh, whole food in its natural state as often as possible.

Don't eat anything your great-grandmother wouldn't
recognize as food.
—Michael Pollan, *The Omnivore's Dilemma: A Natural History of Four Meals*[1]

One evening after physician Mark Hyman had given a lecture, a morbidly obese sixty-year-old man named Samuel approached him. Weighing more than 300 pounds, Samuel asked Hyman if he would be his doctor. Hyman agreed.

During the office visit, Samuel described a life filled with excessive overeating and bingeing; for instance, two cups of heavy whipping cream each night was a typical nightcap. He had a history of extreme yo-yo dieting: losing weight and then gaining it back . . . plus even more. As his obesity worsened, so did his health. By the time Samuel came to see Hyman, he had a plethora of infirmities—profound fatigue, difficulty breathing while walking, stuffed sinuses, swollen legs, severe sleep apnea, dry skin, imbalanced hormones, food sensitivities, and an impaired liver—as well as a wide range of risk factors linked to heart disease, such as diabetes.

What happened next changed Samuel's health and weight, indeed his life, forever: Hyman gave him hope. "I told him that if he did everything I suggested, he would lose weight, feel better, and his symptoms would go away. Everything he had done, he did to himself and could undo," writes Hyman.

What did Hyman suggest? The core of the program he recommended was a diet abundant in nutrient-dense, fresh, unprocessed whole foods (fruits, vegetables, whole grains, beans and peas, and nuts and seeds) "without any restriction on calories or portion size." To enhance Samuel's weight loss, Hyman included a conservative exercise plan of walking slowly, then added interval training once Samuel was in better shape. He also augmented Samuel's fresh-food diet and exercise plan with supplements and herbs that would be helpful in turning around his various ailments. Armed with this advice, Samuel left Hyman's office somewhat skeptical but determined.

After three months on the program, Samuel had lost thirty pounds, his food cravings had disappeared, and some of his symptoms were less severe. Eight months later, "I was shocked when he weighed in," writes Hyman. "He had lost 110 pounds without being on a strict deprivation diet." There was more good news: along with his excess weight, most of Samuel's ailments had vanished or diminished. Just as encouraging, after he had replaced a diet of mostly fast, processed, fat-filled food with fresh, whole, flavor-filled nourishment, what remained was his "continued pleasure in food," writes Hyman. Samuel achieved weight and health success—without deprivation, without restricting calories, and without suffering—in large part because he replaced a predominantly high-calorie, empty-calorie, fast-food diet with a low-fat, nutrient-dense, fresh, and whole-food way of eating that provided the nutrients—in the ratio nature intended—that his body needed to heal.[2]

What was it about Samuel's change from fast food to a fresh, whole-food way of eating that led to such powerful—seemingly effortless—improvements in his weight and well-being? And if it worked for him, might it be beneficial for the millions of us who struggle with the perennial weight-loss question: what's the best diet for losing weight and keeping it off? (Chapter 14, "Introduction to the Recipes: Fresh, Whole, Inverse," will give you optimal-eating guidelines and recipes for attaining and maintaining weight loss and well-being, based on Whole Person Integrative Eating concepts.)

A look at the Fast Foodism overeating style can give us clues about how a diet of mostly fast and processed foods increases your likelihood of being overweight—and, in contrast, how consuming mostly fresh, whole foods—the Whole Person Integrative Eating "get fresh" antidote to the Fast Foodism overeating style—can lead to weight loss and wellness. It's a good idea to become especially familiar with both the Fast Foodism overeating style *and* its remedy, the WPIE fresh, whole food guideline we tell you about in this chapter, because, of the seven overeating styles, our research revealed that Fast Foodism ranked number two as a predictor that you'll gain weight (Emotional Eating, the focus of chapter 6, ranked number one), and Fast Foodism ranked number three as a predictor that you'll overeat.[3] To help you understand more about how replacing the Fast Foodism overeating style with the WPIE antidote of fresh, whole foods, here are some more insights into the eat fresh, weigh less formula we discovered.

The WPIE Training Effect on Fast Foodism

In chapter 1, "Discovering Whole Person Integrative Eating," we told you about the effect our training on Whole Person Integrative Eating had on those who took my eighteen-lesson online course on Whole Person Integrative Eating, and who also filled out both the pre- and post-questionnaire. When Larry and I took a close look at the fast food–fresh food continuum, a distinct eating and weight pattern emerged for both overeating and becoming overweight and obese.

Overeating. Those who ate the most fresh fruits, veggies, grains, legumes, and nuts and seeds were less likely to overeat, while those who reported more frequent consumption of fast (such as McDonald's), processed (canned, packaged), and prepared (deli, takeout) foods— and especially sweets (donuts, muffins) and fried foods (fries, chips, chicken)—were most likely to overeat.

Overweight and obesity. Research participants who consumed mostly fresh, whole foods were more likely to be of normal weight, while those who were overweight, obese, or even morbidly obese ate more processed fast food. In other words, those eating mostly fruits, veggies, grains, legumes, nuts, and seeds were normal weight, whereas those who often ate fast, processed, and prepared foods were more likely to be obese. The biggest weight-gain culprits? Sweets and fried foods were most strongly linked with obesity.[3]

We especially learned a lot about the training effect of Whole Person Integrative Eating on the Fast Foodism overeating style and weight from those who completed the e-course and answered the "What's Your Overeating Style? Self-Assessment Quiz"[4] (chapter 3) both prior to and after taking the eighteen online lessons. Did following the fresh-food guidelines of the WPIE dietary lifestyle lead to weight loss? Absolutely! Over the six weeks, the more people shifted from fast, processed, fried foods to fresh, whole foods, the more weight they lost. (See the appendix, "The Evolution and Science Behind the Overeating Styles," for more about the research on the overeating styles.)

The takeaway: you can up your odds of weight loss and well-being by replacing the Fast Foodism dimension of overeating with the WPIE guideline of fresh, whole food. This chapter will show you how.

Demystifying Fast Food

What is fast food? Some say it's "snack crack." Others call it an "industrial artifact." Corporations proclaim it's a "commodity." From fries and chips to triple burgers and colas, it's the opposite of the "fresh, whole food in its natural state" guideline that Whole Person Integrative Eating suggests as a remedy for the Fast Foodism overeating style.

Fast food typically has five key features: it is often *processed*, with *heated* (often rancid) *oil*, typically *packaged*, and *calorie-* and *chemical-dense*. Most everyone is familiar with fast food, which is inexpensive and prepared and served quickly in restaurants such as McDonald's, Burger King, Wendy's, KFC, and Taco Bell.[5]

Processed food has been cooked, baked, cured, heated, dried, mixed, ground, separated, extracted, sliced, and preserved for a long shelf life. Because processed food is often manufactured, it's typically packaged, canned, jarred, or enclosed in some other sort of container. Fast and processed foods have one thing in common: both are often *junk food*,[6] a slang term referring to fare that's high in calories, salt, sugar, fat, and additives but low in nutrients such as fiber, vitamins, and minerals—hence the term *empty calories*.

What does the Fast Foodism eating style look like? Perhaps a breakfast bar or donut for breakfast; Chicken McNuggets or a burger and a Coke for lunch; and maybe a pepperoni-and-sausage pizza delivered from your nearby pizza parlor for dinner. Add the supersizing of such fast-food staples as burgers, franks, fries, and other food products, such as fried potato chips that are also high-calorie and super-processed—foods often laden with trans fats, sugar, and refined flour[7]—and the alarming increase in obesity should hardly come as a surprise.

With 44 percent of Americans eating fast food once per week, 20 percent twice per week, and 14 percent consuming it three or more times weekly, millions of Americans are indeed living the Fast Foodism overeating style that's contributing to their growing girth. Given these figures, it is also not surprising that the Fast Foodism overeating style is strongly linked with overeating and being overweight or obese.[7,8]

A closer look at the evolution of fast food—and at the ingredients often taken *out* of, and *added* to fast foods—will give you a better understanding of why fast food isn't really food in the traditional sense—it's foodish food, ersatz sort-of-like-food food, but not real food. And we'll explore not only why the modifications that make fast food, well, fast food, can contribute to an expanding waistline but also why, if you're a fast fooder, you're at increased risk for heart disease, diabetes, high blood pressure, certain cancers, and other fast food and diet-linked chronic conditions.[9]

"Takeaways": The Roots of Fast Food

In the 1750s in England, the invention of machinery used in manufacturing (the Industrial Revolution) forever changed the way we make food. No one could know that this development would lead to the fast-food "food products" millions of us eat today. It was the roller mill especially—huge cylinders that could crush and separate the wheat kernel into its elements of flour, germ, and bran—that made the difference.

More than a century later, porcelain mills enabled manufacturers to make white flour (sans the nutrient-dense germ and fiber)—in lieu of whole-wheat flour—inexpensively; ergo, white flour became a popular, easily available staple for the masses. It was called "separated food" at the time because the mill separated the bran, germ, and endosperm (flour) elements of the wheat kernel.

Today we call white flour "refined" or "processed." The health-enhancing "good" fats, vitamins, minerals, antioxidants (which protect body cells from the damaging effects of oxidation), phytochemicals (naturally occurring substances in plant-based foods that have beneficial health effects), and fiber have been processed out of the whole kernel. It has also been refined to have a long shelf life and be easy to use as an ingredient of baked goods that can sit on supermarket shelves for, well, years.

When wheat was being denatured, nutritional science as we know it didn't exist. In the eighteenth century, French chemist Antoine-Laurent Lavoisier had defined the *calorie*, a measure of energy in food, and then in the 1840s German scientist Justus von Liebig isolated proteins, fats, carbohydrates, and minerals in food. But these discoveries were just that—discoveries.[10]

Nothing much changed in the nutrition world until the early 1900s, when diseases of malnutrition such as beriberi and pellagra began to emerge among populations who were consuming "separated grains," meaning that people were developing illnesses due to the processed grains they were consuming, because many nutrients had been taken out. These diseases of malnutrition especially manifested in England and America, where white flour was popular, and in Japan and China, where the population had turned from whole-grain brown rice to milled, processed, denatured white rice.

To combat widespread malnutrition, food manufacturers added back ("enriched") to white-flour and white-rice products the four nutrients we then knew about at the time that had been lost in processing: niacin, riboflavin, thiamin, and iron. This enrichment didn't include fiber or the germ or the more than twenty-five vitamins and minerals we know about now.[10]

Today, to compensate for what's missing, most of the food made by the multibillion-dollar fast-food industry contains more than a few added vitamins and minerals in white-flour products (such as hamburger buns). For instance, to standardize flavor, mouth feel, and a sense of satiety, calorie-rich fat and sugar also have become typical additions.

While fast food alone isn't causing obesity rates to soar (overeating behaviors we've identified,[3] physical inactivity, genetics, the health of the microbiome, and lifestyle all play a part), it plays a key role. In country after country that adopts American eating habits—especially consuming lots of foodish food—obesity increases dramatically.[11] But the opposite is also true. Consider France, where childhood obesity increased steadily for decades due to the adoption of lifestyle habits such as more fast food and less physical activity. What's especially telling (and hopeful), though, is that by 2008—unlike other European countries with *increasing* obesity rates after adopting America's fast food—the trend toward childhood obesity in France had stabilized due to effective governmental policies that promote a healthier diet.[12]

(See Part Three, "Whole Person Integrative Eating Recipes," for more about optimal eating.)

Add-Ins: 4 Weight Boosters in Fast Food

Have you had your enriched white flour, sugar, high-fructose corn syrup, yeast, hydrogenated oil, salt, and wheat gluten today? Or the dough conditioner diacetyl tartaric acid esters of monoglycerides? Or the cancer-linked azodicarbonamide food additive that's been banned in Europe and Australia—but not in the U.S.? If you've had a hamburger at McDonald's today, with ketchup and a Coca-Cola, then, yes, it's likely you've had most or all of the above processed and chemical ingredients . . . and more![13]

In the prior section, we took a look at the health-robbing problems created when food manufacturers began producing food products and stripping food of its original nutrients *in the ratio in which human beings were meant to consume food*. I call what fast-food manufacturers process *out* of food "takeaways." But the ingredients they *add* ("add-ins") to fast, processed foods—I call it "chemical cuisine"—give some clues about why they can put you on the fat—and poor health—tracks.

From fried fish and fries to hamburgers and pizza, the food served in fast food restaurants such as McDonald's, Denny's, and Pizza Hut is familiar to most of us. What may be less well known is that the food is highly processed, prepared in bulk at industrialized central locations, and then shipped to each restaurant.

It's during the processing of fast foods that a seemingly simple item, say white-flour burger buns, becomes high-calorie, high-fat, sugar-laden foodish food. Not only is lots of fat and sugar added, but the *type* of fat that's often used—partially hydrogenated oil—is so toxic to your heart health and waistline that some places, including New York City, have banned its use in restaurants.[14,15] And then there are all those highly processed sweeteners that wreak havoc with your weight.[16]

There are many health-harming additives added to fast, processed, junk food that turn it into what I call "chemical cuisine." And these additives make real food a food *product* that can pose serious weight and other health problems. Even more vital to your health are the four "silent killers" abundant in many fast foods: partially hydrogenated oil, high-fructose corn syrup, toxic chemicals, and increased calories. Let's take a closer look at these four most harmful ingredients.

Partially hydrogenated oil. Unlike polyunsaturated, monounsaturated, and saturated fats that are naturally found in food, partially hydrogenated oil is artificially created when food manufacturers pump hydrogen atoms into liquid vegetable oils (such as corn, soy, and palm) in order to thicken it, enhance flavor, and increase the shelf life of foods (so they can sit on supermarket shelves for years, literally!).

Examples of food products that have been partially saturated with hydrogen atoms to create trans fats include some spreadable, soft margarines and vegetable shortening. When a food or oil is completely—rather than partially—saturated with hydrogen atoms, the result is hard, firm fat, the kind you see in chilled bacon, beef, or butter.

So what's the problem? Why have New York and other cities banned food prepared with partially hydrogenated oils in their restaurants? The partial hydrogenation process creates *trans fatty acids*, commonly called *trans fat*. Unlike polyunsaturated and monounsaturated fats that occur naturally in food, artificially made trans fats pose serious health risks—from heart disease and type 2 diabetes to obesity. Trans fats play havoc with your heart health by raising "bad" LDL cholesterol and triglycerides, lowering your "good" HDL cholesterol, and increasing your risk of blood clots and having a heart attack. The main fast-food culprits containing hydrogenated trans fats: fried and baked food products.

To decrease body fat, one of the best actions you can take is to avoid any food that lists partially hydrogenated oil as an ingredient, because *trans fat makes you fatter than other fats do.* Researchers at Wake Forest University fed the same number of calories to monkeys over a six-year period, with 8 percent of one group's calories coming from olive oil (which is mostly monounsaturated fat) and 8 percent of a second group's calories coming from industrially made trans fats. The monkeys who ate the trans fats gained four times more weight than those on the olive-oil-based diet.

The siren has been sounded against trans fats—loudly—by health professionals nationwide, in Canada, and throughout Europe. The consensus: trans fat isn't safe. If you consume foods containing trans fat, keep your intake to one gram or less. Look at labels. As of January 2006, trans fat is listed along with saturated fat and cholesterol on the Nutrition Facts label of packaged foods in the U.S.

Sugar and high-fructose corn syrup. "Sugar: the ingredient you can trust. And pronounce. There's just one ingredient in real, all-natural sugar: real, all-natural sugar. Plus, it's only 15 little calories per teaspoon. And that's all there is to it."[17] This ad by the sugar industry ran in a local newspaper. Is it accurate? Absolutely. At the same time, though, it hides the whole story: what's hidden is the powerful place sugar takes in the creation of fast, processed foods . . . in huge amounts. Call it *sugar, sucrose, fructose, dextrose, turbinado, amazake, sorbitol, carob powder, high-fructose corn syrup, maple syrup,* or *molasses*—it's sugar. And it's in most fast, processed foods—abundantly.

The ad from the sugar industry said that one teaspoon of sugar is "only 15 little calories per teaspoon. And that's all there is to it." But that's not all there is to it—not when, today, consuming 140 pounds of sugar *per year* is average for most Americans. This is easy to do when just one twenty-ounce serving of processed and sweetened soda, sports drinks, or tea has seventeen teaspoons of sugar—and the average teenager often consumes two of these bottled beverages each day.[18,19] As a contrast, our hunter-gatherer ancestors consumed about twenty teaspoons of sugar *per year*.

Then there's this: much of the sweetener added to fast, processed junk food is in the form of high-fructose corn syrup (HFCS)—which really raises a health alarm, as well as a notch on your belt. Why? When you consume dense amounts of fructose (a form of sugar that comes from fruit) in the super-processed HFCS added to thousands of fast foods and beverages, your brain doesn't recognize that it's a food or that it has calories (energy)—although it is indeed calorie-dense. Instead, your brain thinks you're starving; to compensate, it signals you to keep eating. In other words, HFCS ignites your hunger signals and appetite, and though you're consuming lots of calories, you're still hungry. In response, you eat more . . . and gain more weight.

The HFCS-health story worsens when you consider the ways in which it contributes to more than obesity: this man-made sweetener also increases your risk of heart disease, type 2 diabetes, cancer, and dementia.[19-22] In large part, this assault on our health happens because we're consuming the cheap-to-produce industrial food product HFCS in such large doses, it's comparable to overdosing on a drug or medication that's not good for you. HFCS is absorbed quickly into your bloodstream and liver; in turn, this triggers a spike in insulin, which increases appetite and your odds of gaining weight, diabetes, cancer, dementia, and more. And high doses of HFCS also put you at risk for what's called "leaky gut," meaning it can create small holes in your intestinal lining, allowing bacteria to "leak" into your bloodstream and ignite body-wide inflammation—the root of most chronic conditions.[19]

The takeaway: high-fructose corn syrup is the worst of the refined sweeteners because of the multidimensional ways it can harm your health . . . and waistline.

Toxic chemicals. Azodicarbonamide, calcium peroxide, caramel color made from ammonia, sucralose, monoglycerides and diglycerides, acesulfame potassium, neotame, diacetyl tartaric acid esters of monoglycerides, calcium propionate. And of course, high-fructose corn syrup. These are just a handful of the three thousand food additives approved for use in food in the United States. The rationale? These flavorings, preservatives, colorings, and more are added to food to enhance flavor, extend shelf life, make food look more appealing, and on and on and on.

Packaging materials, too, can be an "indirect additive" because they can add substances to the food they enclose. Consider bisphenol A (BPA), for instance, an insidious compound that is the building block of polycarbonate plastic. Endocrinologist Dr. David Feldman and his team at the Stanford University School of Medicine found that BPA can leach out of the plastic and lining of cans that hold beverages (bottled water, baby bottles) and foods (such as canned tuna) you buy.

What he found was staggering in its implications: even at very low concentrations (10 to 25 billionths of a *mole*, a molecular weight in grams), BPA activated receptor sites of the hormone progesterone, which in turn can increase production of breast cancer cells in humans. In other words, "because of its estrogenic hormonelike properties, BPA has the potential to be important and perhaps even dangerous to people who were eating or drinking out of containers made of this type of polycarbonate plastic."[23]

Since Feldman's breakthrough finding, more than one hundred independently funded studies have added evidence of BPA's harmful health effects. Even at low and short-term doses, exposure to BPA has been linked with increased risk of an alarming number of developmental, neural, and reproductive ailments in infants, children, and adults. A sampling includes breast cancer, prostate disease and cancer, heart disease, stroke, diabetes, hyperactivity, miscarriage, lowered sperm count and sperm defects, and Down's syndrome. And increasingly, BPA is being linked with obesity as well.[24-30]

The evidence linking overweight, obesity, and a plethora of health threats with the ingestion of BPA is so strong that regulatory agencies in Canada have declared BPA "a toxic chemical requiring aggressive action to limit human and environmental exposures," says Frederick vom Saal of the Division of Biological Sciences at the University of

Missouri at Columbia. Studies by vom Saal, the leading researcher on the impact of small concentrations of endocrine disrupters, show that even very small levels of exposure can have huge effects in offspring.[31]

A multitude of studies link not only BPA but also other chemical "outlaws"—phthalates, hexachlorocyclohexane (lindane), pentachlorophenol, DDT, atrazone, dioxins, furans, polychlorinated biphenyls, and some heavy metals, among others—to health threats worldwide.[32]

The takeaway: BPA and related toxins are so harmful to both your weight and well-being, in 2012, the Food and Drug Administration banned it from baby bottles and sippy cups nationwide.[33] But it's still in much plastic and canned packaging. Avoid packaged and canned food products as much as possible, and instead choose fresh, whole foods for optimal health. (This chapter and Part Three, "Whole Person Integrative Eating Recipes," show you how to do this.)

Increased calories. Hydrogenated oil and trans fats, high-fructose corn syrup, and "chemical cuisine" are key players when it comes to putting on pounds, but another major player, unequivocally, is the amount of added sugar and fat calories many Americans consume in the supersized portions offered in our nation's almost two hundred and fifty thousand fast-food restaurants.[34] The arithmetic is easy: large portions of food—especially those that contain lots of high-calorie sugar, oil, and chemicals—are a formula for overeating, large waistlines, and other health-harming side effects.

Clearly, the ingredients in fast food and Americans' love affair with this foodish food have created a deep and multidimensional weight problem in the United States. Though a diet of mostly foodish food plays havoc with our health and well-being, one-quarter of our adult population visits a fast-food restaurant on any given day. We are indeed a fast-food nation with a "chemical cuisine" diet of added hydrogenated oil, high-fructose corn syrup, chemicals, and super-sized calories. The Whole Person Integrative Eating dietary *practice* number three, "Eat fresh, whole food in its natural state as often as possible," is the solution we're suggesting. Here, insights into why fresh, whole food heals and helps with weight loss, and how to integrate it into your life.

Choose Fresh, Whole, Plant-Based Foods

There's a simple way to eat that provides the antidote to the Fast Foodism overeating style. It's a time- and science-tested guideline that has nourished humankind for millennia—and it is how people who are naturally thin—and healthier—eat today. The secret of eating to get slim and stay slim lies in the WPIE Fast Foodism Rx we told you about at the start of the chapter—the way our ancestors ate for thousands of years that allowed humankind not only to survive, but to thrive: *eat fresh, whole food in its natural state as often as possible.*

In Dean Ornish, M.D.'s bestselling, groundbreaking book *Eat More, Weigh Less,* he clearly shows weight loss is not just about *how much* you eat; it's primarily *what* you eat.[34] Actually, what "eat more, weigh less" really means is that if you eat more of certain *types* of food (fresh, whole, mostly plant-based food) instead of focusing on the *amount* of food you eat, you are likely to lose weight. Simply put, calories from fast food and calories from fresh, whole food aren't the same; your body metabolizes real food and junk food differently.

Here, a closer look at the fresh, whole, plant-based foods that lead to weight loss and well-being and scientific studies that support this guideline. In Part Three of this book, the recipes will show you how to put this mostly-plant-based food way of eating into practice each day.

Fruit. An apple a day may do more than keep the doctor away; it may keep you slim. When researchers from the State University of Rio de Janeiro in Brazil put two groups of women on a comparable-calorie diet, those who snacked on an apple lost more weight than those who munched on oatmeal cookies. Why might this be? With an 85 percent water content and lots of soluble fiber, apples are filling; they also keep blood-sugar levels even, which cuts cravings and which signals to your brain that you're full. And because apples are a fresh, whole food, they supply the fiber and nutrients you need in the ratio intended by nature.

Vegetables. Studies have linked abundant mixed salads with weight loss. By "abundant," we mean more than the typical ice-berg-lettuce-and-tomato duo that often passes for a salad in the U.S. Rather, we're talking about a resplendent mix of vegetables that might include lettuces, spinach, and arugula tossed with cherry tomatoes, chopped mushrooms, sliced cucumber, chopped red and green peppers, sliced avocado, beans (such as garbanzos), or baked tofu, a sprinkling of chopped walnuts, grated cheese, and perhaps some raisins.

When researchers at Penn State University studied women who consumed a satisfying salad prior to eating pasta for lunch, they discovered that they ate less pasta than those who hadn't had salad. And there are other weight-loss benefits to both fruits and vegetables: they are the only source of vitamin C. A Purdue University study suggests that vitamin C may be a significant weight-loss aid, helping you to burn fat during physical activity. In fact, this study suggests that vitamin C is a key determinant of weight loss.

Whole grains. Since *whole* grains—that include the germ, fiber, and endosperm—were first cultivated more than ten thousand years ago, they've been a boon to health. Recent research from Harvard University, published in the *American Journal of Clinical Nutrition*, reveals that they also prevent weight gain. In a twelve-year study conducted with more than twelve thousand nurses ages thirty-eight to sixty-three, researchers found that those who ate the most whole-grain foods (such as oatmeal, popcorn, wheat germ, and multigrain breakfast cereal) weighed less than those who ate the least. The difference was quite significant: women in the high whole-grain group had a 49 percent lower risk of gaining weight. (Note: because of what researchers have recently learned about gluten-containing grains and health, consuming *ancient grains*, such as quinoa and amaranth, which have not been hybridized and changed from their original nutrient composition may be a smart choice.)

Legumes. It's a fact. Including dried legumes such as pinto, navy, and lima beans in your diet (not green beans or soybeans) may help you lose weight. When Maurice Bennink, professor of nutrition at Michigan State University, reviewed a plethora of studies on beans published over a twenty-five-year period, he discovered compelling evidence that beans work their weight-loss wonders in three ways:

- Satiety—beans are rich in fiber, so you feel full.
- Sustained energy—beans have a very low glycemic index, and thus glucose is released slowly into the bloodstream, so your blood sugar remains stable.
- Reduced odds of eating calorie-dense fast foods—consuming low-glycemic-index foods tends to lead to subsequent choices of low-glycemic-index foods.

Nuts and seeds. We wouldn't call any kind of high-fat nut a weight-loss food per se, but Harvard researchers found that frequent nut eaters (who consume perhaps a handful of nuts each day) are less likely to gain weight—possibly because nuts are high in protein and fiber, two macronutrients that slow absorption and decrease hunger. And the news gets better: When co-author Dr. Frank Hu, professor of nutrition and epidemiology at the Harvard School of Public Health, looked at results based on nearly one hundred twenty thousand participants in the Nurses' Health Study and the Health Professionals Follow-up Study, he found that those who consumed nuts daily were less likely to gain weight or die prematurely of cancer, heart disease, and respiratory disease. Hu speculates that the composition of nutrients in nuts may be the mechanism by which they help us maintain health.

A balance of nutrients. The naturally occurring nutrients in fresh, whole, lean foods—many that we know about and others that remain to be discovered—not only help to balance your weight and keep you lean but also help prevent, treat, and reverse a plethora of ailments, from heart disease to diabetes. You receive many benefits when you consume food that's as close to its natural state as possible, because fresh, whole, plant-based foods have the whole package of nutrients needed for optimal weight, health, and well-being.

From bioactive compounds and fiber, to vitamins and minerals in fruits, vegetables, whole grains, beans and peas, and nuts and seeds, what fresh, whole, plant-based foods have in common is that their components add up to more than the sum of their parts. In other words, while scientists have isolated particular nutrients in food that are either health enhancing or health robbing, the key to optimal nourishment is *not* to pursue "parts" of foods by turning, for instance, to synthetic, isolated supplements for health and well-being. Rather, nature knows best: follow the WPIE guideline to *consume fresh, whole foods in their natural state as often as possible*, and you'll obtain nutrients in the ratio nature intended. These are the foods that can help to keep you slimmer and healthier.

Recent research on the way in which fast foods versus fresh, whole foods are metabolized in your gut offers still more clues into what to eat for attaining and maintaining weight loss.

Can Gut Microorganisms from Fast Food Make You Fat?

The *microbiome* is the genetic material of all the microbes—bacteria, bacteriophages, fungi, protozoa, and viruses—that live on and inside the human body. A new gut-obesity story is emerging in the world of microbiome research: decades of studies have revealed a strong *association* between the gut microbiome and obesity in humans, but a *cause-and-effect* relationship has been elusive—until now. Rapid developments in the field are showing that the gut microbiome responds quickly and precisely to diet, antibiotics, and other external input in ways that impact a variety of conditions, including obesity and weight management. And the key seems to be the roles of specific sets of gut microbes.

The researchers who discovered the causal gut-microbes-obesity relationship began by conducting what's called a *transplant experiment*: they transplanted various gut microorganisms harbored in the gastrointestinal tract from both lean and obese mice to germ-free mice, meaning mice with organism-free guts. After only two weeks, the mice given the microbiota from obese mice gained more body fat compared to the mice injected with the gut microbiota from lean mice. Clearly, certain gut bacteria were involved in the development of obesity![35]

Knowing that many obese people have what obesity researchers call *Western diet-induced obesity* (DIO), the research team now wanted to know if there was a relationship between gut microbiota, diet—specifically, the fast-food-based standard American diet—and energy balance (high-calorie intake from the Western diet). To find out, they transplanted DIO gut microbiota due to a fast food diet into germ-free mice. Again, the Western diet-induced obesity microbiota promoted more fat gain than transplants from lean donors.[36-38]

Because of such state-of-the-art studies on the microbiome, we now know that the *quality* of the food you eat (fast and processed versus fresh and whole) and your weight are all interconnected. And we also know that gut microbiota—influenced by the quality of the food you eat—is the new unifying factor in the study of obesity.[35-38]

The takeaway: the fresh, whole, plant-based foods we just told you about are what human beings have been consuming for millennia. These foods have the kinds of nutrients (such as fiber, phytochemicals, antioxidants, and so on) that feed "good" bacteria in your gut, which in turn help you to attain and maintain a healthy weight. Think of it this way: Feeding your gut is like fertilizing soil for healthy plants. Tend to your "gut garden" by feeding it fresh, whole foods that will allow it to thrive.

But fill up on fast food replete with processed fats, sugars (especially high-fructose corn syrup), and a motley crew of synthetic chemicals that damage your intestinal lining and feed "bad" bacteria, and you're setting yourself up for anxiety,[39] depression, emotional-eating episodes, inflammation, autoimmune conditions . . . and ongoing weight gain.

Your Fresh-Whole-Food Guide

What exactly are "fresh, whole foods"? They're foods that are real, natural, nourishing, and healthful; their original integrity is intact, and they offer balanced nutrients in the ratio nature intended.

What follows is an easy-to-access primer on plant- and animal-based fresh, whole foods. But first, a caveat:

For Your Consideration

The following foods and food groups are meant as a general guideline only. Avoid any food or food group for which you have a health condition, sensitivity, full-blown allergy, or philosophy that doesn't support consumption.

Plant-Based Foods

Here, a medley of plant-based foods to get you started. Key suggestion: go organic as much as possible in order to avoid toxic pesticides and herbicides. Here are some suggestions to get you started:

Choose:

Vegetables. Dark leafy greens, salad greens, carrots, beets, and cruciferous veggies such as broccoli, cabbage, cauliflower, brussels sprouts, radishes.

Include *fermented, cultured* veggies in your diet, such as sauerkraut, kimchi, pickles, miso, tempeh.

***Whole* pieces of fruit** (instead of fruit juice). Apples, berries (such as blackberries, blueberries, and red berries), cherries, plums, pomegranates, oranges, pears, grapefruit.

***Ancient* whole grains.** Modern wheat is a hybrid descendant of three wheat species considered to be ancient: spelt, einkorn, and emmer. The operative word is *hybrid*, meaning the constituents and nutrient balance of the original kernel have been changed due to technology. Ancient non-wheat grains include bulgur, millet, barley, teff, and oats; pseudocereals are quinoa, amaranth, buckwheat, and chia. If whole grains are part of your diet, consider consuming these ancient options.

Ancient **legumes.** Anasazi beans, adzuki beans, black beans, black-eyed peas, chickpeas, but also pinto beans, kidney beans, red beans.

Nuts and seeds. Raw walnuts, almonds, pumpkin seeds, flax seeds (ground to increase absorption).

Avoid:

Refined, processed grain products. White flour, white rice, white corn, packaged snacks, bread, and refined-grain cereals.

Refined vegetable oils. There are dozens of variations of refined vegetable oils (soy, canola, sunflower, etc.) that have been heated to high temperature so they can sit on supermarket shelves for years, literally. Choose *cold-pressed* oils, and when cooking do not heat oil so that it smokes.

Trans fats and hydrogenated fats. Packaged and processed food products, all fried food.

Animal-Based Foods

Where do fish, poultry, meat, and dairy fit into the whole-food picture? Technically, because they're not plant based, fish, poultry, meat, and dairy products aren't whole foods. Still—if you do eat animal-based food, which most of us do—it's useful to also think of these foods in terms of *fresh* and *whole*. This is because, in general, conventional animal foods contain many environmental pollutants, such as herbicides and insecticides, plus hormones and antibiotics. And because these pollutants are hard for both animals and humans to get rid of, they tend to settle in the liver and in body fat. For damage control, as with plant-based foods, go organic, and avoid animal foods with antibiotics, hormones, and herbicides and pesticides in the feed.

Here are some suggestions to get you started:

Find out if grass-fed beef, free-range poultry, cage-free eggs, or dairy foods that are hormone- and antibiotic-free are available in your grocery store or community.

Choose fresh animal-based food (such as beef, poultry, and wild fish).

Integrate probiotics into your diet for a healthy microbiome. A sampling: unpasteurized yogurt, kefir, raw milk cheeses.

Select fresh-water or wild-caught fish because fresh, wild fish contains fewer chemicals. Avoid farm-raised fish, if possible.

Choose dairy that is free of bovine growth hormone, antibiotics, and other hormones. Consider raw or fermented goat and sheep milk, because these dairy sources are less inflammatory.

Avoid:

Highly processed "products" such as salami, bacon, chicken "nuggets," fried fish, etc.

Animal foods with hormones, antibiotics, etc., plus feed that includes herbicides, pesticides, GMOs, etc.

In other words, the key to optimal nourishment and attaining and maintaining weight loss is to trust that nature is the best nutritionist possible. To reap the rewards—both weight- and health-wise—decide to make fresh, whole food your most-of-the-time way of eating. It's *the* secret to ensuring your mind, body, *and* microbiome will obtain nutrients in the ratio nature intended.

Get Fresh, Weigh Less

Throughout this chapter, I've revealed the ways in which foodish food can make you fat and, conversely, how fresh, whole foods—the foods our ancestors consumed for thousands of years prior to today's chemical cuisine—can lead to leanness (more about this in Part Three, "Whole Person Integrative Eating Recipes").

In other words, to increase your odds of attaining and maintaining weight loss, follow the Whole Person Integrative Eating antidote to the Fast Foodism overeating style we told you about at the start of this chapter: *choose fresh, whole food in its natural state as often as possible.* This means choosing mostly plant-based foods (fruits, veggies, whole grains, legumes, nuts and seeds) with lesser—or no—amounts of free-range, grass-fed dairy, poultry, meat, or wild fish most of the time (see chapter 14, "Introduction to the Recipes: Fresh, Whole, Inverse," for putting fresh-whole-food eating into action). After all, this is how much of humankind ate for thousands of years—prior to the evolution of nutritional science in the twentieth century and prior to what I call *eating by number*, meaning, for instance, counting calories and curtailing carb and fat grams.

The next chapter will give you insights into an overeating style that is likely unfamiliar territory for most of us: Sensory Disregard. In the chapter, you'll discover how to turn the Sensory Disregard overeating style into palate-pleasing adventures that lower your odds of overeating and weight gain while nourishing both body and soul each time you eat.

CHAPTER 9

SENSORY DISREGARD Rx: NOURISH YOUR SENSES

SENSORY DISREGARD Rx

Nourish Your Senses

Whole Person Integrative Eating
Practice #4

Savor and "flavor" food with loving regard.

The truth is that at the end of a well-savored meal both soul and body
enjoy a special well-being . . . the spirit grows more perceptive . . .
—Jean Anthelme Brillat-Savarin[1]

How often do you focus on the aromas, colors, or flavors of food? Do you eat with your senses by appreciating the presentation, "tasting" the textures, or being grateful for the life-giving gift inherent in food? In our research on Whole Person Integrative Eating (WPIE), we found that the Sensory Disregard overeating style is a dependable predictor of overeating and weight gain and that if you're not enjoying your food—indeed, if you're not savoring and flavoring food with love, enjoying food, and infusing pleasure into the dining experience—you're likely to keep eating until you finally do feel a sense of satisfaction.

I told you about making the food-love connection in chapter 1, while I was interviewing cardiologist Dr. K. L. Chopra, father and mentor of integrative medicine pioneer Deepak Chopra, M.D. During our discussion, I lit on Dr. Chopra's comment, based on Hindu scripture from the *Bhagavad Gita*, that "*Prana* is the vital life force of the universe, the cosmic force . . . and it goes into you, into me, with food. When you cook with love, you transfer the love into the food and it is metabolized . . .".[2]

Food and love. The idea so contrasted with traditional nutritional science that it launched my nutrition journey around the world to discover what other world religions, cultural traditions, and ancient Eastern healing systems (such as India's Ayurvedic medicine) had to say about eating with loving regard. When Larry and I put this rich repository of ancient food wisdom together, we discovered the overeating style of Sensory Disregard and, conversely, the ancient-food-wisdom-based guideline of nourishing your senses by both preparing food and eating with loving regard for food, plus taking the time to savor flavors, aromas, colors, and more when you eat.[3]

In other words, we discovered that specific elements of the Sensory Disregard overeating style are powerful predictors of overeating and weight gain, because if you're not enjoying your food—indeed, savoring it and "flavoring" food with loving regard when you eat—you're likely to keep eating until you finally do feel a sense of satisfaction. Indeed, our research revealed that *those who ate the most actually enjoyed their food the least.* This is a staggering finding because it tells us that when you eat with the WPIE guideline of *nourishing your senses*, filled with pleasure and enjoyment of food, you'll likely eat less.

The WPIE Training Effect on Sensory Disregard

Of all the overeating styles we've identified, Sensory Disregard is associated with the *largest number of food-related behaviors we've identified that lead to overeating and weight gain.* Specifically, we identified eighteen statistically significant Sensory Disregard items from our "What's Your Overeating Style? Self-Assessment Quiz"[4] that were closely linked with one another, meaning that if research participants did *not* prepare food with, say, care and appreciation, they were also more likely not to practice other positive elements of this overeating style, such as preparing food with care and appreciation; expressing gratitude for the food before them; experiencing the uplifting feeling of loving regard for the food; awe at the mystery of life in food; savoring the meal with their senses; or reflecting on the meal after eating. (See "The 3 Phases of Sensory-Spiritual Dining: Plan, Dine, Reflect" below for the eighteen items.)

What's key to our findings is this: The 126 individuals who completed the pre- and post-overeating styles quiz[4] after taking the six-week, eighteen-lesson WPIE e-course[5] significantly and substantially improved their scores on each of the eighteen items. It was these research participants who curtailed their overeating and who lost weight.[6]

Overeating. The more research participants implemented *all* eighteen sensory-spiritual items, the less likely they were to overeat. The three sensory-spiritual elements most strongly linked with less overeating were planning meals with care, planning meals with appreciation, and eating with the senses by savoring the scents of food. We also learned that the more participants paid attention to food preparation and eating, the less they ate.[7]

Overweight. Research participants who engaged in the eighteen sensory-spiritual practices of the Whole Person Integrative Eating guidelines of *savoring flavors* and *spicing food with love* were less likely to be overweight. In other words, those who "flavored" their food with the WPIE sensory-spiritual ingredients lost the most weight. (See the appendix, "The Evolution and Science Behind the Overeating Styles," for more about the research on the overeating styles.)

Our findings suggest that you can fill a sense of spiritual emptiness with true nourishment by savoring the flavors in your food and filling yourself with loving regard for the food before you each time you eat. In turn, when you improve your sensory-spiritual relationship with food and eating, you also lower your odds of overeating and becoming overweight or obese.

The sidebar below, "The 3 Phases of Sensory-Spiritual Dining: Plan, Dine, and Reflect," provides all the ingredients you need to practice all the *positive* elements of sensory-spiritual dining. It shows you how to turn Sensory Disregard into the Whole Person Integrative Eating practice of *nourishing your senses* and in turn how to overcome overeating, overweight, and obesity. In other words, it gives you 1) the step-by-step guidelines you need to integrate the WPIE family of sensory and spiritual ingredients, 2) and to practice all the elements of these powerful team members, so you can get the same benefits our research participants did.

The 3 Phases of Sensory-Spiritual Dining:
Plan, Dine, and Reflect

There are three phases of sensory-spiritual dining that can help you nourish your senses—the antidote to the Spiritual Disregard overeating style—each time you eat. Ultimately, the three phases call for integrating the eighteen sensory-spiritual dining elements we have identified into your eating experience before, during, and after eating—as you plan your meal, dine, and then reflect on your eating experience.

Familiarize yourself with the three phases—and then practice each element of sensory-spiritual dining as a path to nourishing your senses and "flavoring" food with love: Whole Person Integrative Eating practice number four.

PLAN: BEFORE EATING	DINE: DURING EATING	REFLECT: AFTER EATING
I plan and prepare meals with:	*I focus on:*	*After eating, I:*
• Care • Appreciation • Blessings	• Surroundings • The food • Color • Aroma • Portion • Flavors	• Savor the moment • Reflect on the meal
	I eat with my senses by savoring:	
	• Presentation • Texture • Scents	
	I appreciate:	
	• The web of humanity that makes meals possible • The elements of nature that create food • The mystery of life in food	
	*I eat with **loving regard** for food.*	

Sensory Delight, Loving Regard

We're especially excited to tell you about the Sensory Disregard over-eating style and its Whole Person Integrative Eating antidote—*to savor and flavor food with loving regard*—because our research is the first to reveal that these sensory and spiritual elements of eating go together like twins. While such an orientation toward food sharply contrasts with the Western model of nutritional science and its eating-by-number relationship to food and eating (counting calories and carbs, figuring fat grams, etc.), the intimate relationship between food, love, and spirituality has been an integral aspect of world religions for millennia.

For instance, as we've seen, the *Bhagavad Gita* espouses infusing food with love, teaching that *prana*, or the consciousness with which food is prepared, is infused into food and in turn "digested" when the food is consumed. Judaism's blessings said over bread, wine, and food bring us into a loving relationship with food and God by reminding us that food is holy. Yogic nutrition guidelines by Swami Sivananda of Rishikesh espouse bringing a loving consciousness to food and meals as an opportunity for spiritual growth.[2] Perhaps our spiritual ancestors discovered intuitively what science is now verifying: there is indeed a spiritual ingredient in the best experiences of food and eating.

What is it like to eat with sensory delight and loving regard? If you've ever looked forward to a special meal—perhaps prepared by a close friend or at a choice restaurant—and you delighted in each forkful of your favorite food—then it's likely you ate while experiencing the color, aroma, flavor, texture, presentation, and portion size of your food. This is *sensory regard*—which is a two-way street: regarding flavors, aroma, colors, etc., leads to focusing on the sensory aspects of food, and a pleasant, sensory-filled dining experience leads to regarding food more.

And if you have ever eaten while reflecting on the mystery of food's ability to sustain life; if you have connected to the way rain, sunshine, wind, air, and soil work together to create the foods that nourish you; and if you have ever filled yourself with loving regard for the origins of the food before you—then you are practicing the Whole Person Integrative Eating antidote to the Sensory Disregard overeating style: *savor and "flavor" food with loving regard*. Your relationship to food is filled with the wonder and delight of eating, and it includes savoring the meaning and mystery of life inherent in your meals. In other words, you are nourishing your senses and flavoring food with love.

Feeding the Senses with the 6 Tastes

Larry and I experienced the power of nourishing the senses, especially with taste but also with the color of food, long before we identified savoring and flavoring food with love as the antidote to the Sensory Disregard overeating style. It was while we were having dinner in a beautiful Thai restaurant, where we'd ordered a salad with which we weren't familiar. Called *miang kham*, the dish that arrived at our table wasn't the familiar American salad of mixed vegetables. Instead, we were presented with a platter that held six small bowls filled with finely chopped and colorful ingredients: lime, peanuts, red onion, red pepper, ginger, and toasted coconut. In the center were a bunch of fresh spinach leaves and a bowl of a very thick and sticky sweet-and-sour paste.

The presentation was enchanting, but because it was also unfamiliar, we asked our waitress how we should proceed. Patiently she showed us how to take a spinach leaf, spread a little paste on it, and sprinkle a tiny portion from each bowl over the paste. Then she created a small food-filled tube by rolling up the leaf. When we tasted the handmade tubular salad, our taste buds burst with flavor. With each bite, an implosion of flavors was released, so much so that we instinctively kept our attention and our anticipation focused on the fantastic flavors and tantalizing tastes that each new bite of miang kham released. (For a miang kham recipe, see "Thai: 5 Flavors of Food" in Part Three.)

With each new bite of miang kham, I thought of the "six flavors of food" that Eastern healing systems—India's Ayurveda, traditional Chinese medicine (TCM), and Tibetan medicine—have espoused for millennia to signal optimal eating and complete nutrition. I had been familiar with the role of the six tastes in Ayurveda and TCM, but I discovered their place in Tibetan medicine during a lecture by Tibetan physician Dr. Namgyal Qusar. In response to a question from the audience about optimal food preparation and nutrient preservation, Dr. Qusar responded by clarifying the Tibetan concept of nutritional balance.

First Dr. Qusar addressed consuming food from all food groups—both plant- and animal-based. Then he added that for complete nutrition, he recommends consuming a meal that includes all six tastes: sweet, sour, salty, bitter, pungent, and astringent. In other words, Tibetan nutrition uses a finely honed sense of taste to ascertain whether a meal is balanced—and to find out, you have to focus your attention on the flavors inside your mouth as you chew.[8]

The six tastes are so integral to health and well-being in Ayurveda that some ancient Ayurvedic schools encourage a sequence of tastes in a meal, progressing from sweet to salty, sour, pungent, bitter, and then astringent.

Our miang kham dining experience was an exceptional example of how fresh food, prepared with care and savored by the diner, can fill the senses and satisfy the soul—two key ingredients lacking in the Sensory Disregard overeating style.

When you take time to experience your food through all your senses—taste (flavor), smell (aroma), sight (presentation), sound (of the surroundings), and touch (kinesthetics)—and to regard the mystery of life inherent in food and in yourself, you're more likely to be truly nourished and less likely to overeat. Dining with your senses (sensory *regard*) and at the same time eating with a deep appreciation for the food before you (spiritual *connection*) are powerful ways to nurture and nourish yourself—and in turn feel fulfilled by the dining experience. When you do this, you're likely to eat less and enjoy food more.

Savoring flavors and bringing a loving sensibility to food and eating are part of a sensory-regard consciousness that has traveled through the centuries via world religions, cultural traditions, and Eastern healing systems. Here, how a ritual of "sacred scents" has been integrated into Judaism's ancient Sabbath ceremony for millennia.

Sacred Scents

Toward dusk on Saturday, after a day of resting, thinking, reading, or playing (just *being* rather than *doing*), the Jewish Sabbath ends when three stars can be seen in the sky. This transition—between the Sabbath and the other days of the week—is celebrated with blessings. Called *havdalah*, meaning "separation," the informal farewell calls for a cup filled with wine, a candle, and a box of spices (*besamin*).

"May the coming week overflow with goodness like the wine in the cup," says the head of the household, holding the *kiddush* cup as it brims with wine. Then comes the lighting of a special candle, made of twisted strands symbolizing the many different kinds of light God has created (the sun, moon, and stars, and the Jewish laws by which to live). Next, a spice box (a replacement for the incense burning of ancient times) is opened, releasing the fragrant scent of cloves, nutmeg, and bay leaves—symbolizing hope for a week that will be pleasant and sweet smelling.

Judaism's brief *havdalah* ceremony signifying the end of Shabbat is rich in the inhalation of sweet and savory spices. Its purpose is to capture the senses and serve as a reminder to hold onto moments of sweetness and peace during the busy workweek. Such symbolism has its roots in the *neshama yeterah*—the second, extra soul Jews are believed to acquire during Shabbat—which enhances the ability to rejoice in tranquility and to live with a feeling of contentment. The holiness and intention of the day is one of *Oneg Shabbat*—the joy, pleasure, relaxation, and ease of the Sabbath.

When Shabbat draws to a close, tradition holds that the extra soul withdraws, leaving the mundane soul in its place. Because it is believed that aromas from the material world are the only aspect that the everyday, remaining soul can enjoy, the spice box and its scents serve to console and connect with the remaining soul throughout the week. In this way, inhaling the sacred aromatics signifies more than the moment of transition from the spiritual to the material world: it also fills our being with the spicy sweetness of each moment. As these sacred scents capture the senses and provide a mindful pause, we are empowered to hold on to the peaceful, meaningful memory of the Sabbath—until next Friday at sunset.[9]

A New Weight-Loss Secret: Feed Your Senses!

Whether it's the scent of freshly brewed coffee, cookies baking in the oven, or warm, toasted garlic bread, delightfully scented food is one of life's greatest pleasures. Our original research revealed that those who eat with awareness of scents in food, plus discernment of flavors and other sensory delights, are less likely to overeat and gain weight.[3] An additional clue that aroma in food can play a part in eating less emerged when Dutch scientists discovered that intensely scented food seems to prompt people to take much smaller bite sizes and consume less throughout the meal.[10] Now a groundbreaking study has taken the Dutch study a step further: researchers in Germany have linked an aroma—specifically, the scent of olive oil—to eating and weighing less.

Olive oil. It's the crown jewel of the Mediterranean diet—long linked with many health benefits, including reducing the risk of heart disease, diabetes, osteoporosis, blood pressure, even breast cancer and weight gain.[11-16] With the latest findings about its aroma, the elixir that is olive oil promises yet other advantages: not only does extra-virgin olive oil increase your sense of satiety, its aroma too may help you stay slim.

Study I: The Olive-Oil-Satiety Link

To make the amazing connection between the scent of olive oil and feeling full, researchers from the German Research Center for Food Chemistry first set out to discover if there were any appetite-suppressing—or -enhancing properties in four different fats: lard, butter, olive oil, and canola oil.[17] To find out, they recruited 120 people, who were split into five groups. Every day for three months, four groups added about two cups of yogurt—enriched with one of four fats—to their daily diet, while the fifth (control) group ate plain no-fat yogurt.

Throughout the study, the subjects were given blood tests, and in this way, the researchers discovered that those who ate the olive-oil yogurt had the greatest increases in serotonin, a hormone that helps you feel full. And because the participants who consumed the olive-oil-infused yogurt felt full, they adjusted their normal caloric intake by eating less—and this simple adjustment kept them from gaining weight. Not so for the canola and lard groups, however, who actually gained weight because they added the yogurt to what they were already eating each day. "You could see that those who felt really satiated reduced their total energy intake," said Dr. Malte Rubach, a nutritional scientist who collaborated with colleagues on the study.[18]

Study II: The Link Between Aroma and Staying Slim

After discovering the link between olive oil and eating less, the German researchers asked this question: might there be something other than the nutrients in the olive oil that led to such different weight outcomes?

To find out, the researchers designed a simple study comprising two groups given nonfat yogurt—but with one difference: the yogurt in one of the groups was mixed with an aroma extract infused with the scent of olive oil. Surprisingly, this one small change made a huge difference in the outcome. Not only did those in the *plain-yogurt group* show lower serotonin levels, they also experienced less satiety after eating the yogurt. And they didn't adjust their caloric intake and therefore consumed, on average, 176 more calories daily.

Meanwhile, those in the *olive-oil-scented group* reduced their caloric intake from other foods, plus their glucose tolerance tests revealed more balanced blood-sugar levels. This matters a lot when it comes to overeating and weight gain, because abrupt swings in blood sugar drive how hungry or satiated you feel. "Our findings show that aroma is capable of regulating satiety," says principal investigator Schieberle.[19] In equally fascinating results, the researchers attributed such stay-slim benefits to *hexanal*, a particular compound that's abundant in Italian olive oils, with a scent that is similar to the scent of freshly cut grass.

Feeding Your Senses:
The Missing Ingredient in Meals

Imagine. Just the smell of olive oil can have a powerful effect on the appetite—so much so that it can help you feel full and cut calories. But there's even more to the scent-stay-slim mystery, for it suggests there's much more to food, weight, and the experience of eating than the conventional calories-in, calories-out formula. Researcher Dr. Rubach explains it this way: "This is the first time where we've really looked at the effects that things other than fatty acids, protein and carbohydrates have on satiety. *Everything that completes our impression of a meal can have an impact* [italics mine]." In other words, "*the physiological impact of a meal is not limited to what (you) can see on the plate* [italics mine]."[18]

We agree—especially because our research too revealed that eating with your senses, preparing meals with care and appreciation, filling yourself with sensory delights and uplifting feelings of gratitude and appreciation while eating, savoring food, and "flavoring" food with loving regard are overlooked aspects of overcoming overeating and ensuing weight gain. With this in mind, we're especially intrigued by Schieberle's research, because it is the first study to confirm that aroma alone may have the power to regulate appetite and in turn be a key tool for overcoming overeating.

Love-Filled Feeding

We just saw that certain scents can influence appetite and in turn reduce overeating. The second part of Sensory Disregard's antidote—eating with loving regard and "flavoring" food with love—may have an even more powerful impact on your health: it may prevent heart disease!

The healing power of eating with loving regard was demonstrated when researcher Robert M. Nerem at Emory University School of Medicine discovered an invisible healing web connecting loving relationships while eating and the metabolism of potentially artery-clogging food. When Nerem set out to learn about the effect diet has on the development of coronary artery disease (CAD), a research assistant on his team fed high-cholesterol bits of rabbit chow to caged rabbits. When it was time to tally the results, team members were confounded: though all the rabbits were fed the same artery-clogging food, some of them had 60 percent less plaque (blockage) in their arteries.

Unable to understand why some rabbits showed early signs of heart disease and others didn't, Nerem and his team retraced each step of the study. Once again, the rabbits in the middle tier of cages fared better than those in the lower and higher rungs. Upon closer scrutiny, the researchers realized that it was the rabbits in the middle tier that the research assistant would take out of the cages to hold, pet, talk to, and play with during feeding. It was harder for the petite assistant to reach the rabbits in the higher and lower tiers, but those in the middle received their food while being held.

Amazed, the scientists repeated the study under much more measured conditions. This time, some rabbits would be fed the high-cholesterol diet while being individually held on a regular basis, while those in the control group would be fed the same diet and be given normal laboratory-animal care but wouldn't be personally nurtured while being fed. Again, the cared-for rabbits showed more than a 60 percent reduction in lesions compared to the comparison group, even though the serum cholesterol levels, heart rates, and blood pressures of all the rabbits were similar.[20]

Nerem's rabbit study suggests that there's a mystery to how we metabolize food, and that the "loving consciousness" we bring to meals makes a difference to how food is metabolized, and in turn it makes a difference to our health. As physician Deepak Chopra said in describing just how powerful invisible nutrients such as loving regard can be to our well-being, "When you look at nutrition from a purely scientific point of view, there is no place for consciousness. And yet, consciousness could be one of the crucial determinants of the metabolism of food itself."[21]

Food Fables to Nourish Your Senses

Bringing loving, sensory regard to food doesn't have to be limited to the meal on the plate before you. Here, two seasonal flavor-food-with-love food fables.

Spring: 2 Edible Flowers Fables

Larry and I were unexpectedly flooded with sensory regard for food—its existence, colors, flavors, and more—during an early-morning springtime trip to our local farmers' market. Our serendipitous, sense-filled culinary adventure began when we learned that flowers—edible flowers, that is—can be part of a palate-pleasing feast. While we were selecting some fresh organic salad greens, our eyes lit on two colorful bins: one filled with red and white rose petals, the other with dainty yellow squash blossoms. Fascinated by the idea of being able to consume—literally—these universal manifestations of springtime, we bought a bagful of each.

Rose-petal sorbet. Feeling joyful and excited by our flower findings, we considered making some rose-petal jam, then instantly turned our attention instead to enhancing and ingesting the spirit of springtime by using pretty, fragrant rose petals as a garnish for some raspberry sorbet (our favorite). Though we knew the petals were pesticide free, we still washed them gently in a bowl of warm water. We then shook some dry, while we used the moisture on the remaining rose petals to attract and hold the confectioners' sugar in which we dipped them.

Squash-blossom bounty. Throughout the week, we continued to celebrate spring each time we savored the subtle flavors inherent in the golden-yellow squash blossoms that we had mixed into the farm-fresh greens or the red rose petals that lingered—ever so delicately—near the raspberry sorbet. With each spoonful of sorbet or forkful of squash-blossom-flavored salad, our hearts smiled at the promise of new life and the bloom of new beginnings that spring brings. And we reflected on the gentle, delicate petals and the feelings and thoughts that often bloom in spring: a sense of hope and optimism, a tug toward new beginnings, and reflections on birth and rebirth. Our hearts were flooded with gratitude and delight each time we thought about or tasted these delicacies.

Autumn: A Golden-Squash-Soup Reverie

For as long as I can remember, I've longed to be in New England during the fall. As the air becomes brisk and the scent of smoke from fireplaces fills the air, the leaves burst with a range of vibrant golden and amber tones that mimic the sunset. For Larry and me, the tones of autumn reflect the transition from the heat of summer to the still grayness of winter—just as the glow of dying embers serves as a bridge from vibrant, hot flames to pallid, pale ash.

Color-rich ingredients. When we're surrounded by the bitter-sweet mood of autumn, we often marvel at the way the colors of this season materialize in food: the deep orange of pumpkin, the golden richness of acorn squash, the earthy brown of chestnuts. Intent on ingesting these marvelous manifestations of fall, we often create some squash soup on the spot. The key ingredients include steamed squash, roasted chestnuts, some fresh tarragon, and chopped scallions. The supporting cast: a mere tablespoon of extra-virgin olive oil; salt and freshly ground pepper, to taste; a bit of brown sugar; and grated fresh ginger—all blended together, then simmered slowly in a miso-based broth.

Our savory soup. As we garnish the golden-squash soup with a flicker of freshly grated nutmeg and a sprig of tarragon, we savor each spoonful and the way the soup makes us feel both grounded and connected to the richness of the earth and the change in seasons. Then, unexpectedly, we feel more than just nourished by the soup; our souls are somehow illuminated by its amber radiance.

Strategies to Nourish Your Senses

The antidotes to the Sensory Disregard overeating style are strategies to nourish your senses each time you eat; they are the WPIE guideline I told you about at the start of the chapter: *Savor and "flavor" food with loving regard.* Here, some simple, practical, but profound strategies to put this WPIE practice into action.

Satisfy your senses. Identify the *colors* of the plate, the utensils, the food, before and while eating. Focus on *scent* in food. Do you like it? Is it whetting your appetite so that you're anticipating that first mouthful? Savor *flavors.* Does the food taste sweet? Sour? Bitter? Salty? Astringent? Pungent?

Experience *textures* of the food—starting with the first bite. With your eyes closed, take a bite of food and begin to chew. Focus solely on the food in your mouth. Can you taste fantastic flavors? Are you able to identify one or more of the six tastes? Simply appreciate every single flavor.

Implement olive-oil ideas. Drizzle extra-virgin olive oil (grass-scented, if available) on a fresh salad made with lots of fresh veggies. Or on toasted, whole-grain rustic bread. Or in a serving of your favorite plain, unsweetened yogurt. Another option: Place a bottle—or small bowl—of your favorite olive oil on the dining table. Inhale and savor the aroma before, during, and after eating.

Infuse food with love. To turn meals into a sensory experience, "eat from a place of spirit," says clinical psychologist Michael Mayer. By this, Dr. Mayer means that when you eat, you access the ancient life force of *chi*. Indeed, when you cultivate *chi*, "you merge with the mysterious energy source in the world that is life itself," says Mayer.[22] When you eat with such heartfelt regard, you make it more and more possible to be satisfied, and in turn you do not need to overeat.

Devout yogis—people who practice yoga—eat "from a place of spirit." They follow a philosophy of *sanatana dharma*, the Sanskrit expression for the underlying, eternal, true essence of all life. Such a philosophy complements the *Bhagavad Gita*, which encourages honoring all living things—including food—as part of an interdependent oneness. When preparing or cooking food, think positive, loving thoughts. Devout Hindus believe such a mentality may be transferred into the food, enhance digestion, and empower the food to nourish body, mind, and soul.

Bring spiritual awareness to food. Earlier I told you about Judaism's havdalah ceremony, which focuses the senses with a "spice box" as a reminder to hold on to the Sabbath's moments of sweetness and peace during the busy workweek. Bringing similar regard to food and the entire experience of dining means you're eating with what in Hebrew is called *Yetzirah*, the spiritual awareness of unity and connection. Consider holding this understanding, recognition, and perception in your heart when you eat.

Savor six tastes. Put the concept of the six tastes into practice. Begin by gathering the ingredients to make the unique leaf-wrapped Thai appetizer-salad called *miang kham* (described earlier in this chapter): one lime, small red onion, and red bell pepper; a piece of ginger; two tablespoons shredded and toasted coconut; some honey (perhaps a quarter cup); and about ten spinach leaves. (Note: The sauce is typically made with finely shredded coconut, ground peanuts, dried shrimp, fish sauce—*nahm bplah*—and some water. The ingredient list for the sauce that is spread on the spinach or green leaf may be intimidating. If so, consider simplifying by using some honey only.)

Chop the lime, onion, pepper, and ginger into tiny pieces. Next, spread a thin layer of sauce or honey (perhaps a teaspoon) on one spinach leaf, then sprinkle a pinch of each chopped ingredient over the sticky honey. Roll up the spinach leaf, creating a small food-filled tube.

Engage your senses as you eat the *miang kham*: sight, touch, smell, taste, and hearing. *Look* at the spinach wrap you're going to eat, and become aware of its texture and color. Is it smooth, rough, light, dark? When you take the wrap in your hands, what does it *feel* like? Is it soft, tough, grainy? Next identify the *smell* of the wrap. Is it sweet? Sour? In between? When you take a bite, do you *taste* one or more flavors? (Hint: the taste of food often changes as you chew.) Finally, how does the wrap you're chewing *sound*? Loud or subtle?

Nourish Your Senses

The antidote to the Sensory Disregard overeating style—nourishing your senses by savoring and "flavoring" food with love—does not require thought or language, just a refocus of your awareness, attention, and intention each time you eat. We have seen that our research on the Whole Person Integrative Eating antidote to Sensory Disregard, and the research of others, suggests that when you develop a meaningful relationship to food and eating by truly savoring flavors and infusing food with loving regard, overeating lessens, and so too does weight.

In other words, you increase the odds of overcoming the Sensory Disregard overeating style by taking the time to nourish your senses each time you eat. Take a closer look at the sidebar, "The 3 Phases of Sensory-Spiritual Dining: Plan, Dine, and Reflect," for a step-by-step guide for turning meals into soul-satisfying, sense-filled adventures.

In the next chapter, "Task Snacking Rx: Mindfulness Eating," you'll discover how Task Snacking can contribute to overeating and increased odds of weight gain. And you'll discover the Whole Person Integrative Eating antidote to Task Snacking—mindfulness eating—plus actions you can take right now to break the cycle of merging eating with other activities.

Eliminating Task Snacking completely isn't necessarily the goal; rather, we'll give you the skills and tools you need to cut down on your food-related multitasking so you can reduce both overeating and your weight. In turn, you'll discover the Whole Person Integrative Eating practice of mindfulness eating—the antidote to Task Snacking and to reduced odds of overeating and weight gain.

CHAPTER 10

TASK SNACKING Rx: MINDFULNESS EATING

TASK SNACKING Rx

Mindfulness Eating

Whole Person Integrative Eating
Practice #5

*Bring moment-to-moment, nonjudgmental awareness
to every aspect of the meal.*

The best way to capture moments is to pay attention.
This is how we cultivate mindfulness.
Mindfulness means being awake.
It means knowing what you are doing.
—Jon Kabat-Zinn[1]

Have you ever meandered through the mall while munching? If so, you're Task Snacking. Do you watch TV, flip through a magazine, or work while eating? These are more task-snacking behaviors. Whatever form it takes—eating a meal or snacking mindlessly while working in front of your computer,[2] driving,[3] watching TV, shopping with a friend, or talking on the phone—the Task Snacking overeating style our research uncovered puts you at risk for becoming overweight.

Consider car cuisine, the growing tendency for drivers to eat in their cars at drive-through restaurants or while driving. As Americans eat more and more meals in their cars, food makers have accommodated them with what they call "cup-holder cuisine": finger-friendly foods and compact meals that are drop-free and glop-free. Examples include cereal bars made with dry milk; a salad in a cup and pancake-like breakfast sandwiches with the yummy taste of maple syrup baked right in (available at McDonald's); squeeze tubes containing yogurt; and drinkable soups that can be sipped from a cup. Some experts say that almost 20 percent of us consume such meals in cars. The "dashboard dining" trend is so entrenched that Honda provides a pop-up table in the console and Saab sells models with refrigerated glove boxes.[3]

As a matter of fact, doing other things while eating is so common in our culture, it's become normal. Not only do most of us not pay much attention to what we're eating and what we're doing while we're eating, but we also don't believe that these Task Snacking eating behaviors have anything to do with our weight. But they do.

The WPIE Training Effect on Task Snacking

You will be very familiar with the seven Task Snacking behaviors we identified that increase your odds of overeating and being over-weight. They include eating while you watch TV, read, work at your desk, work at your computer, ride in or drive your car, and walk or talk on the phone. In the large national sample of 5,256 in-dividuals who took our six-week, eighteen-lesson online course on Whole Person Integrative Eating, their most frequent Task Snack-ing activities were eating while watching TV, followed by reading and working at a desk. People rarely ate while talking on the phone or driving.

Overeating. When we asked whether task snackers tended to overeat, we discovered frequent overeating was linked with each of the seven Task Snacking behaviors. All Task Snacking overeating be-haviors were statistically significant, but only to a modest degree.[4] Still, one Task Snacking item linked to overeating stood out over the rest: eating while watching TV.[5]

Weight. As with overeating, Task Snacking was also linked with weight gain: the more Task Snacking, the more overweight and obesity. The Task Snacking behaviors most correlated with weight gain are eating while in a car, driving, and watching TV.

The bottom line: Ultimately, our research revealed all seven Task Snacking behaviors were slightly to moderately reduced after the six-week, eighteen-lesson e-course.[6] The WPIE e-course helped research participants change their Task Snacking behaviors; in turn, they reduced their overeating, and they lost weight. Those who lost the most weight reduced these specific Task Snacking behaviors: eating while in a car, eating while watching TV, or eating at their desk. The bottom line: less Task Snacking and more mindfulness eating lowers your odds of overeating and increases the likelihood of weight loss. (See the appendix, "The Evolution and Science Behind the Overeating Styles," for more about the research on the overeating styles.)

A Tale of Two Task Snackers

Larry and I vividly remember the moment we realized we were task snackers. We were at Heinrich Heine, a medical university in Düsseldorf, Germany, where we'd been invited to do research on lifestyle (diet, stress management, exercise, and group support) and heart disease, based on Dr. Dean Ornish's heart-disease reversal program.[7] We knew the program well because Larry was Director of Research on the reversal program for more than eighteen years and I was the nutritionist on Ornish's first clinical trial for reversing heart disease.[8]

After several months, when we had become good friends with some colleagues, we heard a knock on our office door around lunchtime. "We're going to the cafeteria for lunch," said Siegfried. "Would you like to join us?" We stopped clicking away at our computers mid-word, put our homemade meal away, gathered our coats, and walked through the wintry campus with three coworkers to the building that housed the cafeteria.

In place of sitting at our desk and working at our computers while eating our lunch, we were greeted by medical students' energetic conversations as they waited in line to choose their food. After our leisurely lunch, convivial conversation, and another chance to walk and talk in the fresh, crisp air, we all returned to work. We would repeat this welcome ritual with our friends many times during the two years we worked in Europe.

Desktop Dining and Weight

Upon reflection, we can't help but think how atypical such a social scenario has become for many Americans. Don't most of us munch mindlessly while working at our desks? One of the first studies to demonstrate the link between eating at your desk (a classic task-snacking behavior) and increased risk of weight gain was done by the American Dietetic Association, which cosponsored a survey with Conagra Foods. When they polled 1,024 full-time employees who worked at desks, they discovered that most ate while working: 67 percent ate lunch, 61 percent nibbled munchies, and 37 percent ate breakfast. An additional 10 percent of men and 7 percent of women, eating their dinners at their desks, continued the habit of Task Snacking into the evening hours.

How might desktop dining translate into an increased risk for piling on pounds? Eating at your desk while working means you're likely to consume more food than you realize, suggests David Grotto of the American Dietetic Association.[2] Along with overeating, staying put also means you're moving less and therefore burning fewer calories than more motion-conscious coworkers. Not surprisingly, this can lead to the tired-but-true formula for weight gain: eating more and moving less.

"That's exactly what happened to me," exclaimed a physician friend of ours when we told him about the link between desktop dining and weight gain. "Because I was on deadline to complete my fifth book, I ate breakfast, lunch, and dinner while working at my computer, between seeing patients," he clarified. "During this time, my wife took over my job of walking our dog each day. After nine months, I finished the manuscript; at the same time, I was surprised to discover I had gained almost twenty pounds. This had never happened to me before." Our health-savvy friend said it took almost a year to get back to his normal weight.

Anatomy of Task Snacking: It's a Double Weight Whammy

It's obvious that if you're a task-snacking couch or mouse potato (you spend lots of time at your computer) it's likely you're not moving much. And this means that, like with our friend who put on twenty pounds while working on his book, minimal physical activity can contribute to weight gain. But so too does Task Snacking. How might Task Snacking work against your waistline when you eat while working, munch while watching TV, or snack while driving? How is eating in a not-too-conscious, not-too-mindful way a recipe for weight gain?

Impaired digestion. Because the brain can attend to only one topic at a time, when you do multiple tasks simultaneously, it constantly shifts its attention. If you were to undergo a PET scan—positron emission tomography is a powerful, noninvasive imaging technique that accurately images the cellular function of the human body—while Task Snacking, it would show lights blinking on and off in areas of the brain associated with the various tasks you're undertaking. When you eat while the mind isn't focused on your food, the digestive process is impaired (see chapters 6 and 8 for more about this), making food not nearly as nutritious as it could be. In turn, this can trigger hunger and the drive to eat more so that you'll feel satisfied via the nutrients your mind and your body need for optimal health—nutrients that you're not effectively metabolizing.

Less satisfaction. Task snacking is a recipe for weight gain in yet another way: when the mind isn't paying full attention to the sensations of food and eating—its taste, scent, texture, presentation, etc. (see chapter 9 for more about this)—then eating itself becomes less satisfying. Put another way, eating while doing other things makes it harder for your mind to register that you are indeed eating. In response, you may compensate for getting less pleasure or gratification from food by continuing to eat more and more.

In other words, you get a "double weight whammy" when you eat while multitasking: when you eat while doing other things, 1) you're impairing the digestive process and how well your body absorbs vitamins and minerals, 2) and you are more likely to overeat because you're not really tasting and enjoying your food and in turn allowing your mind-body to get the message that you're satisfied. When this happens, you may experience food cravings that are really an unconscious signal that you're missing some nutrients in your diet. In this way, Task Snacking can create a vicious cycle of poor digestion, inadequate nutrition, and overeating to try to get the vitamins and minerals you're not metabolizing.

In contrast, there's evidence that paying attention to food while you eat affects how your body metabolizes it in a positive, beneficial way. Because your mind is focused solely on eating, more digestive juices are recruited, starting with saliva. And because eating mindfully slows down the speed with which you eat, you're optimizing the digestive juices in your stomach; in fact, the entire digestive process is enhanced.

The bottom line: mindless Task Snacking may lead to eating more, enjoying it less . . . and gaining weight. What's a task snacker to do? Discover the weight-loss power of mindfulness.

Meet Mindfulness Meditation

In 1979, Jon Kabat-Zinn, Ph.D., put Buddhism's concept of mindfulness on the mind-body medical map when he created the Stress Reduction Clinic at the University of Massachusetts Medical School. Now called Mindfulness-Based Stress Reduction (MBSR), Kabat-Zinn's substantial research on mindfulness meditation over the decades has demonstrated that mindfulness-based interventions improve both mental and physical health.

As with our Whole Person Integrative Eating dietary lifestyle, which integrates ancient food wisdom and modern nutritional science, Kabat-Zinn's mindfulness meditation program evolved when he merged principles from the age-old (fifth century B.C.) philosophy of Buddhism and the five-thousand-year-old practice of yoga with state-of-the-art scientific findings.

What exactly is mindfulness? Says Kabat-Zinn: it is "paying attention, intentionally; an awareness that arises through paying attention, on purpose, in the present moment, non-judgmentally."[9]

What do mindfulness and meditation have to do with Task Snacking, eating, and your weight? A lot. In our research on the seven overeating styles, the more our study participants reduced their Task Snacking and ate more mindfully, the more they reduced their weight.

Some scientists decided to find out more about the mechanisms behind mindfulness and eating and weighing less. Though the field is in its infancy, researchers, wondering if mindfulness can manage weight, have posed these questions: Can a meditative sensibility make a difference to your weight and well-being? And if so, in what way? Here, three studies that delve into the ancient discipline of mindfulness meditation to explore its effect on metabolism and its potential to manage eating disorders, weight, and more.

Metabolism of Mindfulness

Researcher Donald Morse, a physician and professor emeritus at Temple University in Philadelphia, created a unique study to assess whether eating mindfully versus eating while distracted or stressed

(Task Snacking) makes a difference to the metabolism of food. He designed his experiment this way: one group of female college students would meditate for five minutes before eating cereal (a food high in carbohydrates), while another group would distract themselves with mental arithmetic before eating the cereal (a form of Task Snacking). Afterward, when Dr. Morse and his team measured both groups' saliva (where the metabolism of food begins), he discovered that those who meditated mindfully before eating produced 22 percent more of the digestive enzyme alpha-amylase.

Morse's study has two significant implications for task snackers. First, because alpha-amylase helps you digest and metabolize carbohydrates in carbohydrate-dense foods (such as potatoes, bread, and cereal) as well as B vitamins (of which there are eight), if you eat while Task Snacking you're likely to absorb fewer nutrients than you need for your mind-body to function optimally. The study also "shows that there's a real benefit to having a leisurely meal," speculates Morse.[10] "The decrease in alpha-amylase production is just the tip of the iceberg. When you gulp down your food, your entire digestive system is affected."

Morse's study tells us that not only does Task Snacking have long-term implications for your digestion, but his findings also imply that if you make subtle changes in the awareness you bring to food so that you're eating mindfully (doing one thing at a time—eating when you eat, working when you work), you're more likely to stop overeating and gaining weight.[10]

Mindfulness for Managing Binge Eating

Our research on the seven overeating styles tells us that mindfulness and meditative awareness when you eat have a lot to do with your weight: the more our study participants reduced their Task Snacking, the more they reduced their weight—suggesting that you eat less when you focus on your food and the process of eating than when you are Task Snacking. The field of psychology is in the early stages of doing experiments that demonstrate the impact of mindfulness meditation and its link to weight loss, but there are some examples.

In the 1980s Jean Kristeller of Indiana State University, where she is a psychology professor emeritus and the former director of the Center for the Study of Health, Religion, and Spirituality, began to use meditation to help patients de-stress with Herbert Benson, M.D.'s "relaxation response."[18] Then, inspired by Kabat-Zinn's raisin meditation (see the sidebar below, "Raisin' Consciousness," for Kabat-Zinn's mindfulness meditation), she turned her attention to meditation as a vehicle for helping people with compulsive eating problems. Over time she developed her Mindfulness-Based Eating Awareness Training (MB-EAT), a comprehensive nine-week program that integrates the experience of eating with "inner" and "outer" wisdom. The program is replete with meditative exercises that address hunger and satiety, forgiveness, and connecting to the inner wisdom that signals whether you're full and satisfied or hungry, with an appetite for a particular food. MB-EAT focuses on finding satisfaction in quality, not quantity.

To find out whether her MB-EAT program could help women with eating and weight problems, Kristeller recruited eighteen obese women, ages twenty-five to sixty-two. Each met the criteria of the American Psychiatric Association's *Diagnostic and Statistical Manual of Mental Disorders* (DSM-IV) for Binge Eating Disorder (BED), defined as recurrent episodes of out-of-control eating twice a week or more for six months or longer. The intervention focused on three forms of meditation: general mindfulness meditation, eating meditation, and mini-meditations.

With the general meditation, participants were taught to develop focused attention and awareness on an object, such as food. They would do this simply by noting their thoughts, emotions, or bodily sensations, then returning their attention to their breathing when they noticed their thoughts straying. This practice teaches individuals to observe the contents of the mind and the sensations of the body without judgment and at the same time to learn detached awareness. The eating meditation applied the general mindfulness-meditation approach to more specific behaviors, beliefs, and emotions associated with food intake; again, emphasis was on retaining detached awareness. To do the meditation, participants were instructed to take a few moments to stop and become aware of their thoughts and feelings prior to meals or when the urge to binge surfaced.

After learning these techniques, participants met once a week for six weeks. For the first twenty minutes of each session, they discussed their progress and any difficulties experienced during the prior week. Next, they focused on a specific theme related to overcoming binge eating—becoming aware of binge triggers, hunger and satiety, self-forgiveness, relapse prevention, and exercises in eating mindfully. Homework included daily meditation, either directed on tape or self-guided, and mindful-eating exercises.

At the end of the six weeks, Kristeller concluded that the program was indeed beneficial. Three weeks prior to starting the intervention, most women binged an average of five times each week. After three weeks of learning and practicing mindfulness meditation in preparation for the study, the women lowered their average number of bingeing episodes to 3.9. And when the six-week program ended, the average number of binges was less than one (0.9) per week.[11]

Just as encouraging, when Kristeller did a three-week follow-up, she discovered the women were still benefiting, with bingeing episodes occurring less than twice (1.6) weekly. In other words, bingeing behavior continued after the study, but there were far fewer episodes than when the study had started. Significantly, emotions that often sparked a bingeing episode, such as depression and anxiety, decreased. Kristeller's findings were so encouraging that the Center for Complementary and Alternative Medicine at the National Institutes of Health funded the psychologist and her team to do a similar nine-week program to examine how mindfulness meditation can promote weight loss.[11,12]

Ultimately, by practicing mindfulness meditation, the women in Kristeller's study experienced fewer binge-eating episodes. A possible explanation is that when you do mindfulness meditation, you learn to detach yourself from the random impulse to binge and then act on it by eating. It may also mean that practicing mindfulness meditation empowers you to disconnect that circuit in the brain that attaches an emotion with a certain behavior sequence (bingeing).

This suggests that if you have a negative feeling and want to binge, doing mindfulness meditation puts space between your feelings and bingeing; you can realize that feelings come and go and that you don't necessarily have to act on them. You can obtain a sense of control over bingeing and are empowered to turn to it as a coping mechanism less often.

Meditation and Your Weight

A first-of-its-kind study that sheds light on the meditation-weight equation was conducted by researchers at Dr. Dean Ornish's Preventive Medicine Research Institute (PMRI). The study, rooted in work Ornish did throughout the 1980s and 1990s, put meditation on the map by including it as part of a comprehensive program to reverse heart disease through lifestyle changes alone—stress management (meditation and yoga); a no-fat-added, plant-based diet; exercise; and group support—without drugs or surgery. Ornish's research, which has contributed to the medical specialty of lifestyle medicine, was pioneering because it was substantive and sound, and it was published in prestigious medical journals, ranging from the *Journal of the American Medical Association* to *The Lancet* and other peer-reviewed journals.[13,14]

Following the publication of Ornish's reversal research, many health professionals contacted him wanting to know which components of the program contributed the most to reversing heart disease. Was it the low-fat, plant-based diet? The stress-management techniques (yoga and meditation)? Perhaps it was the exercise, or could it be the group support? Or was it the combination of all the components, working synergistically, that brought the benefits? Ornish and his research team decided to find out.

The Multisite Cardiac Lifestyle Intervention Program, designed to study 850 patients with heart disease who had been enrolled in the Ornish reversal program for at least three months, would take a close look at the degree to which changing lifestyle behaviors (diet, exercise, and the stress-management practices of meditation and yoga) could improve risk factors linked with heart disease, such as weight, cholesterol levels, depression, and hostility.[14]

Not surprisingly, results revealed that all three intervention modalities (diet, exercise, and stress management) played a positive role in lowering risk factors for heart disease. For task snackers, though, the most relevant results are three key findings about mindfulness, meditation, and weight.

The first revealed that *the amount of time each person spent meditating was directly linked with the amount of weight lost, regardless of whether participants changed their dietary fat intake or their exercise habits.* In fact, those who did *not* change their dietary fat intake but increased their stress-management practice by as much as six hours per week lost an average of almost twenty pounds for men and more than twelve pounds for women.

Second and equally pertinent, the greatest weight loss was achieved by those who increased their yoga and meditation while they *decreased* their intake of dietary fat. Specifically, those who increased their stress-management practice to six hours per week *and* reduced their dietary-fat intake to 15 percent calories from fat lost an average of about twenty-seven pounds for men and twenty pounds for women at the end of three months.

The third key finding goes against the conventional energy-in (food), energy-out (exercise) guidelines: in the Multisite Cardiac Lifestyle Intervention Program, an increase in exercise didn't contribute any further to the amount of weight loss. Rather, it was *the amount of time participants meditated and the degree to which they lowered their dietary-fat intake that brought the best results.*

Ornish says that practicing all components of his program is the key to achieving beneficial health outcomes—including weight loss. Adds Gerdi Weidner, Ph.D., Vice President of Research at PMRI: "In our analyses, increases in stress management and meditation contributed not only to weight loss but also to reductions in diabetic risk and hostile feelings [a risk factor for heart disease]. And less dietary fat intake added further to weight loss and to reductions in perceived stress."[15]

Why Meditation Works for Weight Loss: A Feel-Good Feedback Loop

Why might the ephemeral, meditative sensibility inherent in the unseeable principles of meditation and mindfulness make a difference to your weight and well-being? The answer to this question has its roots in the growing field of brain research. In one of the first scientific studies on the meditating brain, done in the late 1960s, psychiatrist Gregg Jacobs of Harvard Medical School recorded the EEGs (brain wave patterns) of both meditators and another group of subjects who'd been given books on tape to listen to as a way to relax. Over the next few months, Jacobs noted that the meditators had lower activity in the parietal-lobe section of the brain. When this sensory section of the brain shuts down, it's possible to feel fewer "boundaries" and in turn feel more connected to, and at one with, the universe.[16]

The meditating brain doesn't literally shut down; rather, it slows the receipt of information and keeps it from entering the part of the brain that orients us to time and space. More brain-imaging studies by Richard Davidson at the University of Wisconsin–Madison demonstrated that when you meditate regularly, the brain reorients from a right-prefrontal mindset of stress and discontent to a left-prefrontal disposition of relaxation and joy.[17] This is intriguing in terms of Task Snacking because it explains how your brain produces the relaxation response Herbert Benson discovered among meditators;[18] it is also another perspective about the profound way in which eating mindfully reduces stress and in turn diminishes overeating.

Weidner offers still more possible explanations about why meditation may contribute to weight loss. First, it directs your awareness away from external cues (such as eating lunch at noon, when you "should") to focus your attention internally (eating when you're actually feeling hungry). It may also diminish stress-related eating (discussed in detail in the Emotional Eating Rx chapter)—turning to food when you're feeling anxious or upset. In other words, when you focus your awareness through mindfulness and meditation, you're infusing yourself with a meditative sensibility that quiets the mind, soothes the soul . . . and lowers the odds of overeating linked with Task Snacking.

The Inherent Mindfulness of "Tea Mind"

The Ornish heart-disease reversal program, which includes meditation as a stress-management technique that is linked with weight loss, has its roots in the five-thousand-year-old practice of yoga. Indeed, meditation has been an integral aspect of many cultures, world religions, and spiritual practices for millennia. For instance, so central are a meditative sensibility and refined consciousness to the Way of Tea (*chanoyu*)—often called the Japanese Tea Ceremony—that the concept has infiltrated the language through the centuries with the word *chajin*, describing a person who has internalized the meditative awareness of "tea mind."

I vividly remember the moment I was introduced to the Asian idea of tea mind. It was during a visit to the Urasenke Foundation in San Francisco, where I'd been invited to observe students studying the Japanese Way of Tea. At any given time, I could hear the pouring of water, the clink of the lid on the iron kettle, or the whisking of the powdered green tea in water as it turned into a light, frothy brew. Surrounded by the timeless refinement of *chanoyu*, I realized that as much as it is an actual ceremony, it is also a consciousness, a mentality of elegance, an experiential adventure that unfolds along with the passing moments.

Creating the alchemical brew with this kind of consciousness is a path to tea mind. With roots in Taoism, it means that—like tea—a person's mind is limitless and is a part of everything. Accessing tea mind calls for drinking tea using all your senses, plus awareness of the multitude of practiced steps that have evolved over the centuries.[19,20]

While Taoism provided the aesthetic ideals, it was a Zen Buddhist faction that integrated many Taoist doctrines into Japan's Way of Tea as it is practiced today. This appreciation of aesthetics is evident in the placement of flowers, the profound simplicity of the pottery, the architecture of the teahouse, and of course the tea powder itself.

Practicing tea mind, by observing the visible and invisible elements as they play together to satisfy the senses when you eat, makes you less prone to overeating, in contrast to the busyness and lack of mindfulness inherent in Task Snacking.

Here are some strategies to bring the inherent mindfulness mentality of tea mind into your everyday eating experience—and other actions you can take to bring a meditative, mindful consciousness to meals.

Cultivating Mindfulness

Cultivating mindfulness—paying attention intentionally—empowers you to replace Task Snacking with slowing down long enough to experience the subtleties and health-enhancing benefits of food. When you focus on your food, you're simply tasting it and savoring the experience of eating. Simply put: you're in the moment, and you are simply eating when you're eating.

Here, some strategies for cultivating mindfulness each time you eat—including mindfulness master Jon Kabat-Zinn's classic "Raisin Meditation."

Savor flavor. The next time you eat a meal made with varied ingredients, such as a salad or stew, bring your attention to your mouth; then, as you chew, identify the flavors in your food. Is it mostly sweet, or is salt the major flavor? Did you experience a burst of flavor at the first bite? Are you still enjoying the taste of the food after the second and third bites? For more about savoring flavor and mindfulness, see chapter 9, "Sensory Disregard Rx: Nourish Your Senses."

Move into mindfulness. Here are three distinct steps you can take to replace Task Snacking with conscious, intentional awareness:

1. *Intentionality*: Don't just think about doing it; make a decisive choice to focus on the food before you when you're eating.
2. *Commitment*: Act on your intention. Carry it out by gently letting go of feelings, thoughts, and activities that may be interfering with your intention and commitment to mindfulness.
3. *Focus*: with intention and commitment to mindfulness, keep your attention on the food or food-related activities you are experiencing.

Simply . . . eat when you eat. In other words, focus on all aspects of the eating experience itself—from start to finish—even the cleaning-up process. When you take the time to contemplate food, even for a few seconds before, during, and just after eating, you're taking another step away from Task Snacking and toward making weight loss last. And enjoy!

Raisin' Consciousness

The practice of mindful awareness is rooted in one of Buddhism's earliest sutras, or teachings. Called the Mindfulness Sutra, it describes how to cultivate judgment-free, impartial awareness of what you are doing during each moment.

Jon Kabat-Zinn created what he calls the "Raisin Meditation" so people could have an experiential, hands-on sense of what it means to meditate mindfully. As participants are guided through his Raisin Meditation, they focus on all aspects of the experience of eating a single raisin: how it looks, smells, and feels; what happens in the mouth before, during, and after eating it; the motion and movement involved; the raisin's taste and texture; swallowing; and the role of breathing throughout the experience.

To get the most benefit, first read through the steps before doing the exercise.

1. Sit in a comfortable chair and set a small bowl filled with raisins on a table next to you.
2. Select one raisin from the bowl.
3. Look at the raisin as if it were an alien object you had never seen before. As you look at it, imagine it in its original form as a grape, growing in the sunshine surrounded by air, earth, and water.
4. Continuing to look at the raisin, describe what you see: its texture, color, shape, and anything else that comes to mind.
5. Bring the raisin up to your nose. Smell it. Describe its scent.
6. As you smell the raisin, are you experiencing any changes in your mouth, in your saliva, as you anticipate eating the raisin?
7. How does the raisin feel? Describe it.
8. Become aware of your body and the hand that is holding the raisin. Consider how your hand knows how to hold the raisin, how to bring it up toward your nose.
9. Bring the raisin toward your lips, then place it in your mouth. What motion is your tongue doing? Your jaw? Your teeth? Your cheek?
10. Now focus all your attention in your mouth. Bite into the raisin slowly . . . and begin to chew . . . slowly. Stop after three chews. On which

side of your mouth are you chewing? What are your tongue,
jaw, teeth, and cheek doing now?

11. Describe the taste you're experiencing.

12. Continue to chew, but don't swallow the raisin. Do you notice a
difference in the taste? What is the texture like?

13. Are you tempted to swallow yet? Observe what's happening in your
mouth as you prepare to swallow. Now swallow the raisin. Imagine it
in your stomach, and acknowledge that your body is one raisin heavier.

14. Can you "taste" your breath now? Focus your attention on your
breath as you inhale and exhale slowly.

15. Remain focused on your breath as you continue to inhale and exhale.
Now, simply become silent. If you notice your mind wandering, bring
your attention back to your breath. For the next five, ten, fifteen
minutes or longer, continue to focus on your breathing.[21]

Congratulations! You've just experienced Jon Kabat-Zinn's mindfulness
Raisin Meditation. For the greatest benefit, consider turning each meal or
snack into an opportunity to focus on each aspect of the experience of eating.

Put Tea Mind into Action

Tea mind (see "The Inherent Mindfulness of 'Tea Mind'" above for
more about this) comes naturally from drinking tea and taking time
out of your day to be quiet, still, and observant of your own stillness
. . . and that of the universe. As a path to mindfulness, followers of
Japan's Way of Tea believe that when the elements are balanced and
in harmony, they create a form of perfection. The five elements are
as follows:

- metal (minerals in the soil that help create tea leaves)
- wood (the tea plant)
- water (which brings tea back to life)
- fire (the sun that heats the water)
- earth (the mother of tea and material for teapots)

The next time you sip some tea, bring mindfulness to the experience by thinking about whether you can see and taste each element
with each sip. Consider bringing a similar consciousness to all the beverages you consume during the day.

Mindfulness: The Secret to Overcoming the Task Snacking Overeating Style

To overcome Task Snacking, take a cue from the fifth Whole Person Integrative Eating practice I told you about at the start of this chapter: *bring moment-to-moment, nonjudgmental awareness to every aspect of the meal.* To do this, pay attention to each food-related act, every thought, feeling, and sensation before, during, and after eating. From planning and preparing a meal to serving, eating, and cleaning up, take your actions off autopilot, and instead commit to being fully aware of what your hands, mouth, and mind are experiencing moment to moment—for in the witnessing lies the antidote to Task Snacking and the key to lowering your odds of weight gain.

Welcome to . . . Our Free Audio: The WPIE Guided Meal Meditation

In chapter 13, "In Action: The WPIE Guided Meal Meditation," I'll show you the path to bringing mindfulness to all elements of the Whole Person Integrative Eating dietary lifestyle discussed in Part Two of this book: fresh food, positive emotions, mindfulness, gratitude, love, savoring flavors, pleasant atmospheres, and social connection.

The chapter gives you two options: 1) read chapter 13, "In Action: The WPIE Guided Meal Meditation," 2) or listen to my free eight-minute audio of the WPIE Guided Meal Meditation at least once a day, every day, before eating. To access our free audio, "The WPIE Guided Meal Meditation," visit www.IntegrativeEating.com.

In the next chapter, "Unappetizing Atmosphere Rx: Amiable Ambiance," you'll discover how to overcome the overeating style of Unappetizing Atmosphere through dining by design. We will give you a rich repository of insights and strategies you can use to access the healing power of dining in both *psychologically* and *aesthetically* pleasing surroundings.

CHAPTER 11

UNAPPETIZING ATMOSPHERE Rx: AMIABLE AMBIANCE

UNAPPETIZING ATMOSPHERE Rx

Amiable Ambiance

Whole Person Integrative Eating
Practice #6

Eat in a positive psychological *atmosphere and in pleasant*
aesthetic *surroundings.*

This is an amiable-ambiance food fable—a story of psychologically and aesthetically flavored fare in a snow-laden village high in the Swiss Alps.

It is early on a frosty wintry evening. Larry and I are sitting in a restaurant in Mürren, Switzerland, relishing the respite from the icy chill of the snowy winter landscape outside. We are vacationing, taking a break from the reversing-heart-disease research we've been doing with heart patients at medical centers in both Germany and Holland. Scanning the menu, we're feeling as if we're perched on top of the world in a winter wonderland. Because of the locale and season, we are feeling a subtle sense of withdrawal from the world; it is a time of turning inward.

To get to this Swiss resort town, we took a slow, squeaky tram up the side of a steep, snowy mountain. Because Mürren is so high up and hard to reach, there are no cars here. Instead, the busyness of everyday life is replaced with a special sense of solitude and serenity—and in winter with the opaque, flat, silent quality that comes with snow.

With such winter-inspired feelings in our hearts, we scanned some unforgettable international meals—Swiss, French, Italian dishes—as the powerful scent of a pungent cheese fondue wafted past our table. Mixed-veggie salads and salad with shrimp. Vegetarian strudel with hollandaise sauce. Chicken in blueberry sauce with rice and carrots (a hard-to-find dish in this region of Wiener schnitzel and beef). Veal with mushroom sauce. Or lamb as a main course.

The menu was also resplendent with dessert options—from a blackberry crepe and fresh fruit to artisan cheeses and sorbet. An abundance of some local—but mostly French—wines provided a nice option as an accompaniment to the delightful dinners.

To be truthful, while we recall some culinary delights on menus we scanned that were posted outside of various restaurants, we don't remember much else about what we ate that first night in Mürren. But we do recall—vividly—the feelings, mood, and atmosphere that flavored our dining experience: the soothing serenity of hushed conversation, the cozy comfort of being surrounded by steamed-up windows, the flicker of candlelight on each table, the soothing influence of the scents emanating from the kitchen, and the welcoming warmth of the food we ate. Blended together, all these mood-enhancing ingredients created a particular internal ambiance in both heart and soul as we ate—one that provided a perfect antidote to the icy cold and utter blackness of the moonless winter night that waited for us outside.

Our utterly delightful dining experience in Mürren, Switzerland, demonstrates what it's like to eat in pleasant—exceptionally pleasant— psychological and aesthetic surroundings. In other words, it illustrates what it's like to dine in amiable ambiance—when both your *internal* emotions and the *external* atmosphere are stress free, balanced, and affable.

Eating while enveloped in positive emotions and pleasant surroundings is the opposite of the Unappetizing Atmosphere overeating style we've identified that leads to overeating, overweight, and obesity. In this chapter, we'll focus on the psychological and physical aesthetics of your food life: the atmosphere in your home, in restaurants, and at drive-through restaurants and the *quality* of companionship when you dine with family, friends, and coworkers—or by yourself. At the same time, we'll reveal the influence that unpleasant emotional and aesthetic eating atmospheres have on your mind and body and the steps you can take to turn this overeating style into the Whole Person Integrative Eating practice of eating in a positive *psychological* atmosphere and in pleasant *aesthetic* surroundings.

From Unappetizing Atmosphere to Amiable Ambiance

In chapter 1, I introduced you to Alison, who turned a lifetime struggle with overeating and obesity into a Whole Person Integrative Eating relationship to food that enabled her to attain and sustain weight loss. I am especially reminded of Alison now because after she identified her overeating styles with our self-assessment quiz,[1] she decided the first overeating style she wanted to turn around was Unappetizing Atmosphere.

Her motivation? She knew that spending endless hours sitting in her easy chair in her living room while working at her computer and eating takeout food was a key contributor to her overeating and weight. Not only would an appetizing, pleasing place to eat get her up and out of her chair, it would help her be conscious of her food choices. After choosing the nook in her home that could serve as her "eating oasis," place mats and plates that she found delightful followed. In other words, Alison launched her WPIE dietary lifestyle by creating an amiable ambiance in which to eat. For her, it was a relatively easy overeating style to overcome—with an antidote that brought her instant joy.

Psychological and Aesthetic Considerations

Our research on the overeating styles and their antidote, the Whole Person Integrative Eating dietary lifestyle, suggests that both the *psychological* and the *aesthetic* atmospheres in which you dine hold the power to influence your weight and well-being. What do we mean by *psychological* and *aesthetic atmospheres*? Have you ever eaten in an especially pleasant place, surrounded by supportive people, convivial conversation, and beautiful accoutrements? Perhaps friends took you to a favorite restaurant for your birthday; because they'd organized the meal to celebrate you, the evening crackled with joy, comradery, and laughter.

In the example of the birthday party, your *internal* thoughts and feelings while you eat—likely joyous and happy—determine the psychological atmosphere, while the *external atmosphere* is celebratory and is a source of pleasure. The milieu of your favorite restaurant has an agreeable effect on your psychological state as you and your friends chat over a delicious meal. In response, your heart is open and your soul is singing.

But it's possible your internal psychological state can also be negative, stress-filled, and unpleasant (the definition I use for *stress* is "perceived threat"). Have you ever eaten while feeling frustrated, depressed, or anxious? Or during a disagreement with a colleague? Or while honking at the driver in front of you during rush hour? Or while watching a horror movie or murder mystery on TV? If so, you've had the experience of eating in an unpleasant psychological atmosphere. The surroundings were so hectic or unpleasant that they affected your mind or mental processes in some way—either consciously (when you're arguing with a colleague) or unconsciously (you might not be aware of the impact a horror movie is having on your psyche or digestive process).

The other key component of the Unappetizing Atmosphere overeating style is the *external* aesthetic that surrounds you when you eat. Is the place in which you're dining flooded with overhead fluorescent light and loud music? Are you sitting on a hard plastic bench, eating off damp paper plates? Or perhaps you're eating on the run, grabbing a sandwich from the convenience store as you fill your car with gasoline? These are examples of aesthetically unpleasant surroundings.

As a contrast, envision a place with an atmosphere that's agreeable to you. At a friend's, you're greeted by the aromas of freshly prepared food coming from the kitchen: food your friend has made just for you. Perhaps you take a break from work at your favorite local café to enjoy the brew that the barista makes for you personally. Or soft candlelight makes you aware of a wooden dining table's lovely patina, peeking out from pleasing place mats.

Whether they're appealing or appalling, both the *internal* psychological mood and the *external* physical atmosphere that surround you when you eat may influence how much you eat and the way in which you metabolize food—and in turn your weight and well-being. Here's the research that revealed these new insights into this newly discovered overeating style.

The WPIE Training Effect on Unappetizing Atmosphere

When Larry and I took a closer look at the results from those who took our WPIE online course, we discovered seven unique elements of the Unappetizing Atmosphere overeating style. They are especially distinctive because they describe both the external *physical* atmosphere, as well as the *emotional* environment, which work together either to increase or decrease your odds of overeating and being overweight. The elements comprise eating in a 1) serene, 2) pleasing, 3) fun atmosphere that is 4) relaxing 5) and calm versus eating in a 6) hectic, 7) tense emotional atmosphere. The positive elements that compose this overeating style include *preparing food* in a pleasing, serene, fun atmosphere, while negative attributes involve frequently preparing food in a hectic and tense environment. Two other positive elements are feeling calm and relaxed *after eating*.

Overeating. The interrelated medley of the elements of the Unappetizing Atmosphere overeating style all correlated significantly but moderately with overeating. This suggests that the emotional atmosphere when you are preparing food is related to how frequently you overeat. Research participants overate more often when the atmosphere was negative and unpleasant while preparing food; they overate less often when it was positive.

Overweight and obesity. We found that the link between the emotional atmosphere when you're preparing food and your body mass index (BMI) was significant, but weaker than it is for overeating. This means that although six of the seven elements of the Unappetizing Atmosphere overeating style are significantly linked with weight gain, the link is weak between weight and a negative emotional atmosphere while eating.

Along with discovering the new overeating style of Unappetizing Atmosphere and its antidote, eating in an amiable ambiance, our research revealed it is possible to improve the negative elements of the Unappetizing Atmosphere overeating style after taking the six-week, eighteen-lesson WPIE e-course, and in turn it is also possible to reduce overeating and weight by shifting to eating in an amiable ambiance.[2]

Of special interest is our discovery that feelings of relaxation *after eating* were the strongest predictor of overcoming overeating, followed closely by feeling calm after eating.[3,4] We also found that those who reported preparing food in a more serene and less tense atmosphere were likely to overeat less often.[5] And we found that those who lost the most weight were the people who had fun while preparing food and who felt calm and relaxed after eating.[6]

Such findings suggest that when people change from eating in an Unappetizing Atmosphere frame of mind to eating while filled with pleasant emotions in an amiable ambiance, it can help them reduce both overeating and weight. And it's possible to achieve such success by learning and practicing the Whole Person Integrative Eating dietary lifestyle. (See the appendix, "The Evolution and Science Behind the Overeating Styles," for more about the research on the overeating styles.)

The Unappetizing Atmosphere overeating style, contrasted by its WPIE antidote, eating in an amiable ambiance—such as the dining experience Larry and I had in Switzerland that we told you about earlier—tells us that while food technology and what, how, and where we eat may have changed over the years, the emotions and kinds of surroundings that nourish our soul have not.

What happens to your mind-body when the atmosphere in which you eat reflects the Unappetizing Atmosphere overeating style—when it is a milieu that is jarring to the psyche? When both the psychological and the aesthetic surroundings aren't just unwelcoming and unpleasant but overtly hostile? An unusual study done just after World War II offers insights.

Hostile Ingredients

On June 16, 1951, the prestigious medical journal *The Lancet* published a study that couldn't be done today. Not only were children involved, but the conditions were so health threatening—both emotionally and physically—that a modern-day review board would never approve the study design. In 1948 British nutritionist Elsie M. Widdowson was working at orphanages in Germany, where thousands of children had lost their families in World War II. It was a time of extreme trauma for the orphans, and their suffering was exacerbated by food shortages and rationing.

While working at two orphanages, Widdowson was able to observe and record an extraordinary situation that evolved. Her one-year study started when she decided to monitor and measure the impact of additional servings of food on the children's weight and height. Would those who received extra food gain more weight than those who received rations only? Would they grow taller than children who ate less? To find out, during the first six months Widdowson gave children at both orphanages equal food portions; during the second six-month period she fed children at one orphanage larger portions of bread, jam, and orange juice. Throughout the twelve months of the study, she weighed and measured the height of the children every ten days.

When she looked at the height and weight charts, Widdowson was perplexed. During the first six months, when everyone received equal portions, children at one orphanage had gained a lot more weight and had grown much more than children at the other orphanage. Things became even more confounding during the second six-month period, when the children who had been fed *more* food gained *less* weight and height than the others.

Widdowson pondered whether it was possible for children to thrive—or not—regardless of the quantity of food they ate. But when she scrutinized the atmosphere in both orphanages, she got an unexpected explanation for the seemingly contradictory results: Frau Schwarz. The children who had failed to gain weight and grow had been overseen by a strict disciplinarian who chose mealtime to publicly ridicule and rebuke some of them. This explained the difference. "By the time she had finished," wrote Widdowson, "all the children would be in a state of considerable agitation, and several of them might be in tears."[7] Coda: when Frau Schwartz supervised another wing of the orphanage, the same dynamic occurred. Children who were upset and agitated during meals failed to thrive.

Have you ever felt hungry, then lost your appetite because you were upset? Or did your food "sit like a lump" because you'd eaten while agitated? Perhaps you've eaten to stuff down feelings (see chapter 6 for more about this). The idea that your psychological state can influence digestion is now so familiar that it's easy to lose sight of how amazing Widdowson's findings were considered. But amazing they are. The discovery that children's psychological state when they eat can be so powerful that it can actually determine whether they gain weight, grow, and thrive is remarkable—and it leads to the question of how our internal thoughts and feelings and the external environment influence the way we metabolize food and in turn our weight and health.

Some scientists have explored the role that your emotions and eating environment can influence how your body metabolizes food. What they found is quite amazing.

Discovering the Stress–Poor Digestion Link

One of the most remarkable stories of how emotions can affect digestion starts in 1822, on Mackinac Island in Michigan, when an army surgeon named William Beaumont treated eighteen-year-old French Canadian fur trapper Alexis St. Martin for an accidental gunshot wound to his stomach. Shot at close range, St. Martin was so seriously injured that Beaumont didn't expect him to survive. Not only did St. Martin live but the major wound healed, except for a small opening in his stomach.

At the time, little was known about the process of digestion; it was a mystery discussed in the medical community in Europe, especially France. Ignorant of the debate that raged but intrigued by the puzzle of digestion, Beaumont turned St. Martin's mishap into groundbreaking observational studies: over a period of ten years, during which time he performed about 200 experiments, he became the first medical scientist to observe and carefully record a human being's digestive process.

What exactly occurred when food was digested? What were the elements of stomach acid? Beaumont documented it all. He was the first to show that digestion actually slowed down when someone was upset. How did this come about? Because Beaumont's observational studies were time-consuming and difficult—unpleasant and difficult to endure—St. Martin would become irritated. For instance, the only way Beaumont could observe digestion was to place food via a silk string into the opening in St. Martin's stomach and then remove the string to observe any changes. And it was during one of these experiments that Beaumont observed that the food wasn't digested as well when St. Martin was upset.[8]

Since Beaumont's pioneering observations, science has made great strides in decoding the emotions-and-digestion puzzle—what behavioral scientists today might describe as the mind-body connection. They've answered the question "Why does it matter if you eat while stressed or when you're experiencing unpleasant emotions?" (which was what happened to the children in Widdowson's experiment who failed to prosper).

Though there are many definitions of stress, here I'm defining it as a perceived threat to either physical or emotional well-being. When you eat while stressed, your brain releases a torrent of sometimes-contradictory hormones (chemical messengers) that put your digestive system in disarray. For instance, to give you strength for fight or flight in response to a perceived threat, your body may manufacture the fat-friendly hormone cortisol or CRH (corticotrophin-releasing hormone), which in turn produces energy-giving adrenaline. CRH can also suppress your appetite (what seems to have happened to Widdowson's upset orphans), or it may have the opposite impact: it may produce steroids (organic fat-soluble compounds) that can make you hungry—and prompt you to overeat calorie-dense foods such as cookies, cake, or potato chips. In other words, whether the source is internal or external, an unpleasant psychological atmosphere can cause your body to produce hormones that prompt you to eat more.

Mealtime Emotions and Your Weight

Why have we been created with an amazingly strong connection between the brain and the digestive system—a relationship so powerful that the stomach and intestines are abundant in nerve cells, even more so than the spinal cord? Why has our mind-body been designed to pay such close attention to our internal environment, meaning our thoughts and emotions, as well as our external surroundings—with the ability to respond accordingly? Mind-body medicine pioneer and neuroscientist Candace B. Pert, who discovered the opiate receptor, the cellular binding site for feel-good endorphins in the brain, provides some insights.[9]

Pert's pioneering work presents a scientific picture about how environment may influence digestion and increase the drive to overeat: in other words: stress more, eat more. The story starts with substances called peptides, which reside not only in the brain but throughout your entire body. And it is neuropeptides specifically that act as the biological foundation for the awareness we bring to meals—indeed, to all aspects of our lives.

What's unique about neuropeptides is that they are released into the bloodstream by nerve cells. The link to nerve cells is fascinating because the hormones and other chemicals made by your mind-body create a two-way freeway that serves as a dynamic information network between the brain and the digestive system. Neuropeptides influence your experience of your world, and vice versa: your consciousness—or mind, thoughts, and emotions—affects your biology. Put another way, your body is strongly influenced by your emotions. Because of this, "the environment in which you eat has a lot to do with your emotional experience at mealtime," writes Pert. Eat in an unappetizing emotional or physical atmosphere, and "it's a kind of disintegration, a mind-body split that will lead to *weight gain* [italics mine] and disease conditions caused . . . by incomplete digestion."[10]

But there's another reason you're likely to eat more and gain weight when you consume food in an unpleasant *external* atmosphere: it also influences the quality (worse) and quantity (more) of food you eat. Researchers discovered this when they asked thirty subjects to watch *Love Story*, a sad movie that leads people to cry easily and often. As the study subjects watched the film, they ate 28 percent more buttered, salty popcorn (124.97 grams versus 97.97 grams) than they did while watching *Sweet Home Alabama*, a breezy comedy.[11]

The same researchers found similar results with college students asked to read about children who died in a fire. As they read the heart-breaking news, they ate four times more M&M's than raisins from nearby bowls of snacks. In contrast, when the same students read about a delightful chance reunion among four old friends, they didn't turn to unhealthful food but rather to healthful snacks.[11] The message: if you want to eat less and weigh less, refrain from using the dinner table as a place to argue or scold or think about unpleasant things.

From Food and Fuel to Optimal Healing Environments

Plenty of situations lend themselves to creating unpleasant and discordant psychological and aesthetic eating atmospheres. Consider this common scenario. Imagine you're driving in Anywhere, U.S.A., and you pull into a gas station. When you get out of your car to fuel up, a sign tells you that you need to pay inside. As you walk past other motorists filling their tanks, you cringe slightly as you register the potent smell of petroleum.

Feeling a bit queasy from the odor, you walk inside to prepay. Your nostrils are instantly filled with the scent of rancid cooking oil; at the same time, the harshness of the overhead fluorescent lighting causes you to squint a bit. While waiting in line, you glance at the TV on the counter, which is blasting bad news. You're also privy to a distasteful discussion between the cashier and the customer in front of you, who claims he's been shortchanged. You look around to locate the source of the unappetizing aroma and realize it's coming from a fast-food outlet that shares space with the gas-station store. You notice a customer eating a hamburger and fries as he walks out the door toward his car. He'll probably eat while driving, you think as you continue to wait.

Were you aware of the subtle assault such an atmosphere was making on your psyche and the way it was impacting your digestive system, your weight, your entire being?

Although it's still an emerging field, the medical community is becoming more and more aware that environment has a profound impact on health and healing. In response, the Optimal Healing Environments movement is gaining momentum. For instance, at the second symposium on Optimal Healing Environments, more than fifty scientists and clinicians were invited to define *healing environments* and challenges related to creating them.[12]

Given our own research on Whole Person Integrative Eating and the discovery of the Unappetizing Atmosphere overeating style we have identified, the work of Marc Schweitzer and colleagues especially captured my attention, because it identified elements that are integral to a healing environment: personal space; sound or noise; temperature; fresh air and ventilation; enjoyable social interaction (social support); warm, natural light; color; a view and experience of nature; arts, aesthetics, and entertainment (such as music).[13]

Throughout the day, you have plenty of opportunities to eat in environments that can nourish both body and soul. Even better, create your own nourishing dining atmosphere whenever possible.

Crafting Amiable Eating Atmospheres

Most of us know that eating in congenial surroundings is, at the very least, enjoyable. This is good news since you can access or create delightful surroundings anytime. Envision a fall picnic, for instance, surrounded by the colors of the season in the leaves and in the deep orange of pumpkin soup. Or think of the soothing comfort of a homemade stew eaten in winter as candlelight flickers. To increase your odds of achieving and maintaining optimal weight, here are some suggestions for creating affable psychological and aesthetically pleasing dining milieus as often as possible.

Cherish china. When Oprah did a show on "anti-aging breakthroughs," a weight-loss lifestyle was one of the topics. To highlight the elements of her successful weight loss, an audience member shared her personal success story. Along with moving more and choosing fresh food, she created an aesthetic atmosphere as part of her twenty-two-pound weight loss. "I put my portion [of food] on beautiful plates, with great style, lovely linens, crystal, [and] china, and enjoyed every morsel," she said. "No more standing in the kitchen eating out of a little container." Whenever possible, eat on quality plates with your best utensils, and sit down at a dining table to enjoy your meal even more.[14]

Release negative emotions. Thanks to Candace Pert's research on emotions and digestion, it's safe to say that the psychological atmosphere in which you eat influences the way you metabolize food and in turn your weight and well-being. That's why you'll find it helpful to release toxic molecules of emotion when you eat. If you find yourself ruminating about something unpleasant, put your emotions on hold and press the pause button as you eat; instead, think about something agreeable. You can always return to the problem later. Or, if the people with whom you're dining are more negative than positive, try to redirect the conversation by asking them to share something that's working well or is enjoyable in their lives.

Rest, relax. A friend of ours who is a yogi told us that after she shared a large lunch in the home of a revered family in India, her hosts invited her to lie down and rest so that she could digest the meal in a peaceful and quiet environment. In a time- and work-driven country such as the U.S., this isn't a realistic option, but what we can do is a modified version: after eating, take the time to enjoy some easygoing conversation with others, relaxing music, or an interesting article.

Walk away. A friend of mine told me that not too long after she read our research paper on the overeating styles,[15] she was feeling hypoglycemic (weak from low blood sugar) and hungry in the middle of the day while "choring." She made the spontaneous decision to buy a sweet from a gourmet cookie shop to quickly appease her hunger. But she was dissuaded from staying by the acid-rock music that blasted from speakers and by the uninterested clerks who talked among themselves instead of taking her order. She found a friendlier place down the block for a midday munch. When you eat out—whether it's a full meal or a munchie—choose an amiable place whenever possible.

Limit lighting. One of our favorite restaurants has low-hanging lights above each booth, which we find harsh (although good friends of ours from Germany like this lighting a lot because they enjoy having a good view of their food). Each time we eat there, we think about how much more we'd enjoy the meal and the entire dining experience if instead it were infused with candlelight. When you eat at home, consider diffusing the light by turning on a nearby lamp, dimming your overhead light, or adding candles near the food in front of you.

Eat outside. If you have access to a park near your house, outdoor dining tables and chairs in the courtyard where you work, or a café that enables you to eat outdoors, take advantage of the opportunity to enjoy fresh air and beautiful surroundings—weather permitting, of course! And there's another benefit: you can get a little exercise while walking to your favorite outdoor eating place.

Dine by Design

When our research showed the Unappetizing Atmosphere overeating style was linked with overeating, what astonished us was that, as with all the overeating styles, it was statistically significant, meaning that it's not due to chance that when you eat in an Unappetizing Atmosphere, you're at increased risk for overeating and weight gain.[15]

The bottom line: dining in psychologically and aesthetically pleasing surroundings can be a powerful determinant of your weight. Commit to "designing" the most pleasant ambiance possible each time you eat. And integrate the sixth Whole Person Integrative Eating practice we told you about at the start of the chapter into your everyday life: *Eat in a positive* psychological *atmosphere and in pleasant* aesthetic *surroundings.*

In chapter 12, "Solo Dining Rx: Share Fare," you'll discover the overeating style of Solo Dining, and you'll learn how dining alone most of the time can contribute to overeating. To counteract the Solo Dining overeating style, we'll show you how dining with others can be a balm for body, heart, and soul. And we'll give you the "ingredients" and skills you need to create enjoyable dining experiences with others. As your eating shifts from a "me" mentality to a "we" awareness—and, more and more, as you share food and the dining experience with others—you'll be taking yet another step toward fulfillment and curtailing overeating.

CHAPTER 12

SOLO DINING Rx: SHARE FARE

SOLO DINING Rx

Share Fare

Whole Person Integrative Eating
Practice #7

Enjoy food-related experiences with others.

One of our most memorable meals with others was a dining experience Larry and I had one New Year's Eve that was cradled in hospitality, friendship, fresh food . . . and an ancient heart-to-heart ritual. It all began when we met Nailia Menne at our friend Roslyn's home in northern California. Originally from Kazakhstan, Nailia told us about the *tamada* tradition when I mentioned that the English language needed a new word to describe the invisible ingredients that create "meal magic" when friends share good conversation while enjoying delicious food.

"There is an ancient tradition that no Kazakh celebration is complete without wine and a *tamada*, the host or toastmaster, whose role is to create a pleasurable ambiance and ensure that everyone present is honored and enjoys the occasion," Nailia told us.

"Whether the gathering is small or a meal for many, it is a great honor for the person who is asked to be the tamada. Throughout the meal, starting with the elderly, for whom there is much respect, followed by those who have traveled far for the occasion, the tamada invites each guest to toast people, the food, or the event. From the first course to the main course and then dessert, the *tamada* invites a toast. In this way, every person is honored through the modern expression of an ancient tradition that embodies the best of friendship and shared food."

As New Year's Eve continued to unfold, I knew that not only had I found the word for a time-honored ritual that embodies the special spirit of shared food and friendship but I had just had the honor of having experienced this heart-to-heart, meaningful, love-filled tradition.

Before continuing to explore the healing power of Social Nutrition, I'd like to make a toast to you, dear reader: this chapter is dedicated to tamada-flavored food and friendship . . . for everyone . . . all ways, all days.

A Solo Dining Culture

At the start of a presentation or workshop, I sometimes begin by inviting participants to share a memorable meal. At first, there's often silence and stares. Then, slowly, I see a few raised hands as more and more people recall an outstanding dining experience. Here's a sampling of some shared-meal memories: a homemade holiday feast at the home of lifelong friends; savoring simple campfire food as a preteen during an overnight with girlfriends; a romantic anniversary meal at a candlelit restaurant, savored by an elderly couple who found each other late in life.

In my experience, shared reveries of cherished meals *always* include eating with others in warm, welcoming, pleasing surroundings—and often the other elements of the Whole Person Integrative Eating dietary lifestyle: fresh food, positive feelings, gratitude, mindfulness, and loving regard. I don't recall hearing a memorable meal story that reflects the "Solo Dining" overeating style: eating a sandwich or snack, perhaps while texting or being otherwise distracted by the details of daily life; driving home at night while munching a five-hundred-calorie muffin from a nearby convenience store; or having a secret, private "zone out" in front of the TV with a pint of ice cream and a bag of chips.

Do you see yourself in any of the above new-normal Solo Dining overeating experiences? If so, you have lots of company. We are a lonely culture, and nowhere is this more evident than in the millions who eat meals by themselves. Children reach for a piece of packaged pizza, then eat it at the computer; single working women heat up their low-cal frozen meal in the microwave, then dine solo while watching TV; and anxious traveling salesmen are driven to dashboard dining while en route to yet another meeting.

Not surprisingly, these Solo Dining scenarios also reflect the other overeating styles: Food Fretting, Task Snacking, Emotional Eating, Fast Foodism, Unappetizing Atmosphere, and Sensory Disregard. After all, the seven overeating styles are an interconnected family of eating behaviors that lead to weight issues (see chapter 2 for more about the overeating styles). Here are insights we gleaned from our research on Whole Person Integrative Eating when we took a closer look at the Solo Dining overeating style.

The WPIE Training Effect on Solo Dining

As with all the overeating styles, we found that Social Nutrition too is an interconnected family of eating behaviors, though the connections are somewhat weak: 1) eating with family, 2) eating with friends, 3) eating alone, 4) and eating at home at the dining table. This means that when people eat at home and at the dining table it is natural to find that they also typically eat with family and eat by themselves less often.[1]

Overeating. A closer look at the Social Nutrition elements from our national sample of 5,256 revealed that those who eat at home at the dining table are less likely to overeat and to be overweight. Eating at home at the dining table was the strongest predictor of less overeating and weight gain. Eating with family or eating alone didn't have any relationship to overeating or weight.[2]

Weight loss. When we asked the sample of 192 individuals who filled out both the pre- and post-overeating styles questionnaire[3,4] after taking the WPIE e-course[5] about their social eating behaviors, again the element of "eating at home at the dining table" stood out. The more the research participants increased their frequency of eating meals at home at their dining table, the more weight they lost and the less they overate. And though the connection was weaker, eating more frequently with family and friends was also linked with weight loss.[6] (See the appendix, "The Evolution and Science Behind the Overeating Styles," for more about the research on the overeating styles.)

But this is not the end of the Solo Dining story. We want you to know that our findings about the Solo Dining overeating style are limited by the fact that when we first developed the questionnaire, we asked only a few questions about Solo Dining. Because of this, as our Whole Person Integrative Eating program evolved, so too did our overeating styles questionnaire. The "What's Your Overeating Style? Self-Assessment Quiz" in chapter 3 is our revised, updated, more complete version of the quiz, including more Social Nutrition elements—as is the interpretation of your score at the end of the quiz.[3,4] We also want you to know that the quiz in this book is statistically validated—meaning that you can depend on it to provide accurate insights into your personal overeating styles, and the items in the questionnaire provide steps you can take to overcome them.

Still, what's sobering about our research findings on Solo Dining is the discovery that chronic social isolation while eating increases the probability that you'll overeat.[1] Our research suggests this, and so does a growing body of state-of-the-art studies from many researchers worldwide. Here, a look at the latest research on the new-normal Solo Dining trend and what it means to your weight and well-being.

Solo Dining, Loneliness, and Obesity

If you typically eat alone, you've got lots of company. The statistics on the Solo Dining overeating style are nothing less than daunting. As far back as ten years ago, surveys revealed that the eat-alone trend was escalating: 30 to 40 percent of families were not eating together most of the time.[7] Hoping to make inroads into traditional, social, sit-down family meals, the Centre for Fathering launched "Eat with Your Family Day" in 2003.[8] Still, today, nearly half—46 percent—of adults are completely alone when they eat.[9]

Indeed, the escalating eat-alone trend is a growing concern, with more and more studies supporting our discovery about the Solo Dining overeating style and its link to being overweight and obese. Still more researchers are finding links between the Solo Dining trend, its twin, loneliness, and being overweight and obese.[10,11] A sampling:

- Researchers in Japan found that eating alone and living alone are jointly associated with higher risk of obesity and unhealthy eating behaviors (translation: consuming lots of fast, processed junk food) in both men and women.[10]

- In a U.S. study with 8,459 kindergarten children, those who watched TV during dinner—instead of eating family meals while having convivial conversation—were more likely to be overweight by the time they were in third grade.[12]
- A two-year study out of Korea revealed that the obesity rate of those who ate all three meals—breakfast, lunch, and dinner—by themselves was 1.4 times higher than those who ate all meals with others.[13] Yet another study from Korea showed a clear correlation between lone diners in their twenties and their being obese.[14]

While the new-normal eat-alone trend may seem quite disheartening, please keep in mind that whether you eat alone—or with others—it is part of a web of the Whole Person Integrative Eating antidotes to the overeating styles, meaning that whether you eat with others or solo, it is one of seven elements of Whole Person Integrative Eating. This means it is simply one of the chords of the food-and-dining symphony and its relationship to your weight and well-being. In other words, people who typically eat by themselves may or may not practice the other overeating styles. For instance, unlike the people in the study from Japan, who lived alone and ate mostly fast food and gained weight, it's possible to eat alone and typically choose fresh, whole food and therefore not necessarily overeat and gain weight.

There's also this to consider: I interpret the discouraging data about escalating Solo Dining, loneliness, and their link to weight gain as an opportunity, a chance to make small social changes while eating that have the potential to lead to big mind-body health and weight benefits. The section below, called "Recipes for Social Nourishment," offers insights into initiating and integrating meaningful person-to-person interaction with acquaintances, friends, coworkers, or family members over a cup of coffee, a snack, or a full-fledged meal once or more throughout the day. These social "recipes" give you some ideas about steps you can take toward social nourishment and weight loss.

The following studies about social nourishment provide still more insights into the healing power of eating with others versus the relatively new phenomenon of Solo Dining and its link to overeating, overweight, and obesity.

Study I: The Healing Power of Social Ties

The idea that family meals can serve as a buffer against ailments emerged in a landmark twenty-five-year study that began in the early 1960s in the small town of Roseto, Pennsylvania, when a local physician told researcher Stewart Wolf that he rarely saw cases of heart disease in the town's Italian American population. Intrigued, Wolf set out to study the Rosetans, hoping to discover why their rate of heart disease was so low. Even though they consumed a traditional high-fat, high-cholesterol Italian American diet of sauces, sausages, and other artery-clogging food, the rate of heart disease and mortality from heart attacks remained low in Roseto.

As the long-term study progressed, so did the rate of heart disease among the Italian Americans—so much so that it soon equaled that of the general American population. When Wolf and his colleagues scrutinized the data, the main difference that surfaced was the change in human relationships. When the study started, close family ties and community cohesion were the norm; it was common to find three generations living together in one home. But as the children became adults, they moved away from Roseto. Over time, family and community cohesion began to weaken, along with commitment to religion, relationships, and traditional values. The close-knit way of life that had united Rosetans since their migration to Roseto in 1882 had ended—along with its prophylactic effect on heart disease.[15]

Social connection. When a meal is infused with social ingredients, some kind of healing alchemy seems to be set into motion. Indeed, the Roseto study suggests that eating in a socially supportive atmosphere can serve as a buffer against ailments.

The Roseto study explores the shift in heart disease of an Italian American community over a quarter century, but it is also about the influence of human relationships and social support on the metabolism of high-fat, high-cholesterol, calorie-dense foods. Amazingly, this study suggests that when social support is present in our lives, especially when we eat, *what* we eat—even foods not perceived as being heart healthy—is somehow metabolized differently and in turn may not harm health.

Study II: The Healing Power of Love-Filled Feeding

Research results on the people of Roseto seemed to have anticipated future studies that would serendipitously link dining with others in a caring, supportive environment to health and healing benefits. For instance, in chapter 9, "Sensory Disregard Rx: Nourish Your Senses," I told you about an amazing study by researcher Robert M. Nerem at Emory University School of Medicine, who, as with the Roseto social study, discovered an invisible healing web between caring relationships and the health-protecting metabolism of potentially artery-clogging food. Recall that rabbits in the middle tier of cages fed a high-cholesterol diet—who were held, talked to, and nurtured during feeding—fared better in terms of clogged arteries than those in the lower and higher rungs.[16]

A Perspective-Taking Moment

Both the Roseto and the rabbit studies imply that there's a mystery to how we metabolize food and that eating while experiencing a pleasant, caring connection to others matters. Physician Deepak Chopra speculates about such invisible nutrients in food with his statement that "consciousness could be one of the crucial determinants of the metabolism of food itself."[17]

The studies we've looked at in this chapter on the power of caring social interactions while eating versus the effect of Solo Dining and loneliness on the metabolism of food suggest that social support impacts the way our bodies use our food—so much so that it has the power to halt the development of heart disease.[15,16] Or it can influence whether we gain weight . . . or not.[6,10-14] Call it awareness, realization, or perception, the "consciousness" to which Chopra alludes implies a special sensibility—an invisible, hard-to-measure mystery—that somehow plays an essential and critical role in the metabolism of food itself. And when this consciousness is miraculously activated, not only does it have the power to neutralize the metabolism of potentially artery-clogging cholesterol and fat that we've consumed, but it also can protect us against becoming obese.[1,2,15,16,18]

Such insights provide further support for the Whole Person Integrative Eating antidote to the Solo Dining overeating style we're suggesting in this chapter: *enjoy food-related experiences with others.* The Roseto and rabbit studies tell us that this WPIE practice is more than just words or a generic guideline to follow; rather, state-of-the-art science is telling us that enjoying food with others may provide a path to overcoming overeating and overweight and other conditions linked to a "lonely heart."

What follows are some recipes, literal and figurative, for starting your own Social Nutrition traditions by turning a table for one into a table for two, three, or more.

Recipes for Social Nourishment

Columnist and cookbook author Marion Cunningham has described Solo Dining and the other new-normal overeating styles we're telling you about in this book as "a motel life"—going in, going out, then grabbing something to eat alone. "When you eat this way, you don't create deep connections," said Cunningham, "and you miss the opportunity to get to know about the people you're living with when you don't sit around the table and share yourself around food," she told me during an interview.

"We're fed more than food when we eat with others. Instead of taking a solitary trip through life, when you dine with family you learn to share and care for others, as well as social skills, tradition, and ritual. Talk begins to flow, feelings are expressed, and a sense of well-being takes over."[19] Such is the nourishment that beckons when we reset the American table.

Below are some suggestions for turning Solo Dining into an experience filled with social delight, pleasure, and nourishment.

Set a friendship-flavored table. To imbue a meal with a soul-satisfying connection to others, consider orchestrating a café get-together or hosting a dinner at your place, then asking one special friend to ensure everyone is honored and enjoys the occasion by serving as the *tamada* toastmaster—the tradition we told you about at the start of the chapter. In this way, you and your friends are creating your own tamada ritual that encourages a welcoming and memorable dining experience for all. And now I'd like to make a *tamada* toast: to friendship-flavored food.

Make an old family recipe. Create your own multigenerational meal memories. Start a family tradition by inviting one or more family members over to enjoy a meal made using a recipe from an older member of your family—perhaps an aunt or uncle, parent, or cousin. Launch each meal by setting a glowing table with special ware.

Create a cooking club "family." Invite coworkers, friends, and community members with whom you interact—a librarian, neighbors, people who work in restaurants—to be part of your cooking club "family." Rotate meals at the homes of members. In the spirit of *tamada*, share meal memories and stories as you dine.

Savor family-and-friend food. Consider placing a picture of a family- or friendship-filled dining experience on the table as you eat. If your mother used to make a special meal that you particularly enjoyed, make it for yourself on a weekend and freeze it, then let it defrost while you're at work one day so you can enjoy it when you get home. As you enjoy the special memory-filled dish, reflect on your family members or beloved friends as you eat.

Collect family recipes. Prior to the latter half of the twentieth century, the recipes parents made for their families were often learned from *their* parents or other family members. Create your own culinary family tree and a connection to your food roots by putting together a collection of family recipes.

Have a multigenerational meal. Make a favorite recipe and then invite friends and family from different generations to come for an informal meal.

Create quick-fix family fare. If you're time pressured but you enjoy planning activities in advance, this is a unique way to create a family meal. Pick a day, set aside some time, and plan your meals for the week. Shop for ingredients and prep them all in advance, then place the prepped food in the freezer. When it's time to have one of the meals, both you and your family can assemble the ingredients and cook them together as the need arises. Voilà! Dinner is served.

Dine with your pet. If you have a dog or cat or bird or other pet that you love, consider enjoying a beverage or eating a meal at the same time that your pet eats.

Share a memory meal. Enjoy food with friends and family members even when you're dining alone. Just prior to eating, think of a family member, friend, or other person you admire or love, living or not. Eat your meal while holding their memory in your heart.

Choosing solo dining. There may be times when you simply need some solitude while eating. When you choose Solo Dining, consider eating in silence while focusing on your food. Close your eyes and then inhale and exhale slowly. Throughout the meal, eat from your heart (see chapter 7, "Appreciate Food," for tips for eating from the heart and connecting to food while you eat).

Enjoy Food-Related Experiences with Others

The antidote to the Solo Dining overeating style? Take a cue from the *tamada* tradition of honoring each person at the dining table, the heart-disease-protection power gleaned from the Roseto social study, and the eating-while-cared-for rabbit study: holding regard for those at your dining table, share your food experiences with others. As often as possible, enjoy a fresh meal, snack, or beverage with coworkers, family, or friends. In other words, follow the remedy for the Solo Dining overeating style by integrating the seventh Whole Person Integrative Eating practice into your everyday meals: *enjoy food-related experiences with others.*

I understand. As simple as the solution to the Solo Dining overeating style may seem, I know it can be a challenge to implement, given the demands of busy schedules and cell phones, pagers, and e-mail that can keep us on call twenty-four hours a day. Still, perhaps the ancient social message in food writer Marion Cunningham's wisdom that "we're fed more than food when we eat with others" is worth considering: "It is one thing to eat," she said; "it is another to dine on lovingly prepared food with good friends."[19] For when we do, not only is our appetite sated but body, mind, and soul too are nourished.

In the next chapter, "In Action: The WPIE Guided Meal Meditation," you are cordially invited to experience *all* the elements of the Whole Person Integrative Eating practice. As you'll see, the WPIE guided meal meditation I created empowers you to infuse both yourself and your food with all the notes of WPIE discussed throughout this section: fresh food, positive emotions, gratitude, mindfulness, loving regard, pleasing ambiance, and social connection.

As you practice implementing the seven principles of WPIE more and more, you're replacing each of the seven overeating styles with a dietary lifestyle that nourishes you physically, emotionally, spiritually, and socially . . . and lowers your odds of overeating and being overweight or obese.

CHAPTER 13

IN ACTION:
THE WPIE GUIDED MEAL MEDITATION

To receive the most subtle particles in the food, you must
be fully conscious, wide awake, full of love. If the entire system
is ready to receive food in that perfect way, then the food
is moved to pour out its hidden riches . . . when food opens
itself, it gives you all that it has in the way of pure, divine energies.[1]

—O.M. Aivanhov, *The Yoga of Nutrition*

"The quality of one's life depends on the quality of attention," writes
Deepak Chopra in *Ageless Body, Timeless Mind*.[2] So too are your weight
and mind-body well-being strongly influenced by the "quality of attention" you bring to food and eating. Not only may giving quality
attention to each element of the Whole Person Integrative Eating dietary lifestyle ward off weight but it also holds the power to balance
emotions, digestion, the absorption of nutrients, blood-sugar levels,
and more.

Welcome to the WPIE guided meal meditation. As you practice
integrating each ingredient more and more, you'll become empowered to experience food as the symphonic masterpiece that it is, that
plays the notes you need to overcome the overeating styles by replacing them with the elements of the Whole Person Integrative Eating
(WPIE) dietary lifestyle: fresh food, positive feelings, mindfulness,
gratitude, sensory and loving regard, amiable ambiance, and social

connection. Another helpful distinction is this: I created the WPIE Guided Meal Meditation to empower you to turn Whole Person Integrative Eating into an actual *practice*, a health-enhancing relationship to food and eating . . . for life.

Meet Ancient-New Meditation

Meditation. In the East, yogis say it leads to a super-conscious state that emerges from the cessation of thought; Taoists tell us it helps "to come into harmony with all things and all moments";[3] while believers of Zen Buddhism present it as a path to sudden illumination.[4] In the West, meditation has more often been linked to the mystical and monastic. For instance, the *Cabala*, a Jewish mystical teaching, turns to it to carry consciousness through various "gateways," while early Christian monks and saints used meditation as a stringent contemplative process to achieve spiritual exaltation.

A tradition for thousands of years, the word *meditation* comes from the Latin *meditari*, which implies "deep, continued reflection, a concentrated dwelling in thought."[5] But while it is often linked with the concept of contemplation, it may also involve emptying the mind by eliminating *thoughts* from consciousness (*apophatic* meditation) or holding a specific *image, idea*, or *word* in the mind's eye (*cataphatic* meditation).

Whether the source of meditation techniques comes from ancient Eastern or Western traditions—or the more modern trend to merge meditation techniques with mindfulness to manage stress—the goal is the same: to enhance relaxation and self-awareness and to suffuse the mind, heart, and soul with a sense of unity, union, and connection.

The WPIE Guided Meal Meditation

The *intention* behind our Whole Person Integrative Eating Guided Meal Meditation is to show you how to use a meditative awareness to connect to food and eating in the WPIE way so that you nourish body, mind, and soul each time you eat, and in the process you up your odds of losing weight and keeping it off. Achieving such success calls for creating a conscious connection to all elements of the Whole Person Integrative Eating dietary lifestyle we've been telling you about in this section of the book.

Here are the key steps you'll need to practice, internalize, and integrate the WPIE Guided Meal Meditation into each eating experience.

Getting Ready:

Review the WPIE Meal Meditation that follows, while keeping in mind I created it so you can internalize, apply, and benefit from each element of the Whole Person Integrative Eating dietary lifestyle each time you eat.

- **Just before eating, position yourself** the same way each time you dine. For instance, perhaps you may prefer to fold your hands gently in your lap, or to rest them on the table.
- **Now simply relax** by inhaling deeply, then exhaling slowly. Do this three times. Inhale to the count of five; exhale to the count of eight.
- **Put the world on pause.** *As you weave together the moments of the WPIE Guided Meal Meditation, the rest of the world must wait.*

The Meditation:

- **Visualize.** While looking at the food before you, envision a ball of golden liquid light several inches above your head. Then imagine the golden liquid melting, then flowing through the top of your head (the crown *chakra*, or energy center), and then throughout your arms, hands, torso, legs, and feet.

Meet Mudras

Symbolic hand gestures used during meditation, called mudras, have stood at the center of meditative awareness for ages. In the practice of yoga, for instance, mudras are used with the intention of drawing yourself inward and channeling your body's energy flow.[6] The intention of the mudra used in the WPIE Meal Meditation is to direct energy from both your heart chakra, or energy center, and your hands to your food.

- **Create a mudra.** Continuing to envision golden light throughout your body, position your hands as if there were a small beach ball hovering just over your food and your hands are holding that beach ball. As you hold your hands above your food, envision rays of the golden liquid light emanating from your heart center (chakra) and hands into the food before you.
- **Choose fresh, whole foods.** Holding regard for food in your heart, focus on what you are eating. Is the food in front of you fresh and whole? Does the meal include fresh, whole plant-based

foods (vegetables, fruits, whole grains, beans and peas, nuts and seeds)? Or lean fish, poultry, meat, or dairy? Or is it fast food and processed? In other words, have you taken the time to choose food that is a positive life force, a nurturer, a gift that recharges and sustains? (See chapter 8, "Fast Foodism Rx: Get Fresh," for more about this.)

- **Tune into feelings.** Continuing to relax and breathe deeply, identify how you are feeling. First, are you feeling hungry? And if so, how hungry: a little, somewhat, or a lot? Use this knowledge to make a decision about how much or how little you want to eat. Also, are you filled with positive emotions and loving regard for food? Or do you need to release negative feelings—such as anger and anxiety—before eating? (See chapter 6, "Emotional Eating Rx: Positive Feelings," for more about this.)

- **Craft amiable ambiances.** What are your *external* psychological and aesthetic atmospheres? If you're with people, is there tension? Arguing? Anger? Or are people talking, laughing, and enjoying themselves? What kinds of sounds surround you? Are you—and your surroundings—calm and quiet? Or are you—and the people around you—distracted and busy? Continue to focus on both the psychological vibe and your surroundings throughout your meal.

- **Practice mindfulness.** Eating mindfully—paying attention, intentionally—includes bringing a meditative awareness to all elements of the WPIE dietary lifestyle. Consider: Is the food before you nourishing . . . or not? How are you feeling? Is the external environment pleasant and welcoming? Are you holding gratitude and loving regard in your heart? Be aware of the colors, fragrance, and flavor of the food. Is there a lot of food? Or not? Are you eating with, or thinking about, people you like?

- **Be appreciative.** Continuing to hold the imaginary ball over your food, while remaining calm and relaxed, feel appreciation for the food before you. Consider expressing your gratitude with a *mantra*—a word or sound that you repeat that aids concentration or mindfulness—either silently or verbally. This could be a blessing or prayer. Or simply say thanks for the food in front of you.

- **Practice sensory regard.** The WPIE Meal Meditation also includes bringing loving regard to food and being aware that your senses play an important part in the experience of the WPIE dietary lifestyle. Look at the food in front of you. What colors do you see? Is the fragrance and flavor of the food sweet or sour? Is the food hot, warm, or chilled? Continuing to hold the "beach ball" mudra over your food, and envisioning golden rays from your heart and hands to your food, "flavor" your food with loving regard.

- **Unite socially.** If you are dining with others, envision a ray or thread of the golden liquid connecting your heart center to the heart center of the other person or people at the table. If you're alone, connect the golden thread to a memory of a person, or people, with whom you've enjoyed memorable meals.

- **Infuse food with loving regard**. The WPIE Guided Meal Meditation calls for evoking loving intention, filling your mind-body with loving regard, and then projecting it onto the food. To do this, focus again on the golden energy flowing through you. As your hands continue to surround both sides of the dish, visualize or project rays of the golden light into your food. In this way, you "flavor" both yourself and your food with loving intention.

Now, feeling relaxed and calm, with awareness of your *internal* (feelings, appreciation, mindfulness, loving regard) and *external* (the food, physical surroundings, social connection) environments, with a sense of loving connection in your heart and nonjudgmental attention on your food, it is time to begin the extraordinary experience of eating.

Free Audio: The Whole Person Integrative Eating Guided Meal Meditation

You are invited . . .

I created a free audio of the Whole Person Integrative Eating (WPIE) Guided Meal Meditation so you can reap the weight-loss rewards of all the WPIE elements each time you eat. This chapter—indeed, this entire book—shows you how to do this. So too does my eight-minute WPIE Guided Meal Meditation. Listen to it at least once a day, every day, before you eat. Or download the audio and then listen to it as often as possible, until you know it well enough to do on your own. To access our free WPIE meal meditation, please visit "The WPIE Guided Meal Meditation" at www.IntegrativeEating.com.

Practicing the WPIE Guided Meal Meditation

Each time you practice the WPIE Guided Meal Meditation—either by reading this chapter or listening to the free audio, "The WPIE Guided Meal Meditation," you'll be metabolizing the ultimate multivitamin, one that holds the power to lead to weight loss, but also to nourish your physical, emotional, spiritual, and social well-being.

As you get better at weaving together each moment of the WPIE Guided Meal Meditation, consider using it whenever you're involved in any food-related activity—from planting and harvesting to planning a meal, shopping, eating, clearing the table, digesting, or doing dishes. Over time, you'll discover that by practicing the WPIE Guided Meal Meditation, you may overcome the overeating styles and access food's invisible power to sustain, rejuvenate, and nourish.

Part Three, "Whole Person Integrative Eating Recipes," is the next section of this book. As with our research on Whole Person Integrative Eating that we told you about in Part One, and all the elements of the WPIE dietary lifestyle described in Part Two, the recipes and guidelines in Part Three are also based on a distillation of ancient food wisdom that is supported by modern nutritional science. The key concepts you'll discover in the recipe section, which have traveled through the centuries, are highlighted in the title of the next chapter: "Introduction to the Recipes: Fresh, Whole, Inverse."

PART THREE

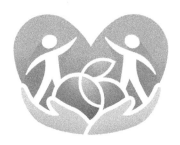

Whole Person Integrative Eating Recipes

CHAPTER 14

INTRODUCTION TO THE RECIPES: FRESH, WHOLE, INVERSE

Eat food. Not too much. Mostly plants.
—Michael Pollan, *In Defense of Food: An Eater's Manifesto*[1]

If you've ever wondered if there's a clear, simple, scientifically sound solution you can trust to the what-to-eat conundrum to lose weight and keep it off, there is! And it's *not* the latest diet du jour; indeed, it's not a diet at all. Rather, it's the what-to-eat guideline of the Whole Person Integrative Eating dietary lifestyle we wrote about in "Fast Foodism Rx: Get Fresh": return to your food roots—to the ancient food wisdom on which humankind not only survived but thrived for millennia[2-4] and which today's modern nutritional science is recommending over and over again as the nutritional path to health and healing:[5-7] *eat fresh, whole foods in their natural state as often as possible.*

But this chapter is about more than the fresh-whole-food guideline. It is about a "new" way of eating that has been around for thousands of years; a way of eating I call *inverse eating* that can help you stop the slide into obesity and its family of related conditions—if you integrate the time-tested recipes in this chapter into the other elements of the WPIE dietary lifestyle. For you to better understand what I mean by *ancient-new inverse eating*, let's first take a brief look at where we are now, food- and weight-wise, and why it's the opposite of inverse eating.

Where We Are Now

In chapter 8, I told you about Fast Foodism, one of the seven overeating styles we've identified that's typical for millions of Americans;[2] indeed, for more and more people worldwide. As you may recall, many develop weight problems because typical American Fast Foodism fare focuses on foods that aren't fresh, whole, and lean; rather, they're highly processed, packaged foods replete with lots of calories, health-harming unnatural fats, denatured white flour, and sugar—plus processed meats such as salami instead of free-range, lean, grass-fed chicken or beef.

Indeed, if plant-based foods are in our diet at all, they're likely to come in the form of french fries, ketchup, baked goods (made with white flour and lots of added fat and sugar), roasted, salted, and fat-laden nuts (such as peanut butter with added trans fats), or a sprinkling of lettuce (usually iceberg) that we flavor with bottled dressing high in fat, sugar, and calories. And if we do choose whole-grain bread, a close look at the label reveals it's often laden with unwanted additives such as HFCS or partially hydrogenated oil. In other words, most of us eat lots of processed dairy, poultry, meat, fish, and grains with occasional (if any) servings of fresh, whole fruits, vegetables, whole grains, legumes, nuts and seeds.

If you think the Fast Foodism way of eating is an exaggeration, consider this: 93 percent of the fast-food standard American diet (SAD) consists of highly processed, often chemical-, fat-, and sugar-laden food—while 7 percent of the "vegetables" most Americans manage to eat is mostly ketchup and fries.[8-10]

And then there's this: if you're a fast fooder, you're also much more susceptible to a plethora of other life-threatening, diet-related conditions—from heart disease, diabetes, and high blood pressure to depression, ongoing inflammation, certain cancers, and more.[11-14] In other words, if your primary diet is foodish food, with lots of chips, sweets, colas, processed meats, fried chicken, canned fish, and dairy—with little or no fruit, veggies, legumes, whole grains, nuts and seeds—your dietary lifestyle is threatening more, much more, than your waistline.

What can you do to stop the slide into obesity and its family of related conditions? Here, the number-one simple step you can take to lose weight and keep it off: eat inversely—mostly plant-based foods with smaller or no portions of animal-based foods. It's a new yet old way of eating that's been around for thousands of years! Let me explain.

Meet Inverse Eating

Whether you're looking at the traditional diets of Mediterranean, Asian, South American, African, Indian, or Native American cultures, they all have one way of eating in common: meals are mostly plant-based foods (fruits, veggies, grains, beans and peas, and nuts and seeds), with lesser amounts of animal-based foods (dairy, fish, poultry, and meat). In other words, the diets of most cultures worldwide are— and have been for thousands of years—mostly plant-based foods as the *centerpiece* of the meal, and animal-based foods as a *condiment* or side dish.

Clearly, this is the *inverse* of the almost 40 percent—approximately 84.8 million Americans—who eat fast food every day[15] and the 91 percent—at least 290 million Americans—who completely miss the mark of meeting the U.S. dietary guidelines of a half to two cups of vegetables per day. Same with fruit: only 12 percent of Americans consume one-and-a-half to two servings per day.[16] In other words, most Americans eat the standard American diet of mostly processed animal-based foods with few, or no plant-based foods.

With SAD as a starting point, I use the term *inverse eating* to describe the *antithesis*, or inverse, of the standard American diet: the opposite way of eating that evolved naturally over thousands of years and includes mostly fresh, whole, plant-based foods supplemented with small, occasional servings of fresh (meaning chemical-free), whole (meaning that the initial constituents of the food are intact), grass-fed, free-range poultry and meat; *wild* fish (not farm-raised); and hormone- and antibiotic-free dairy foods. (Please see chapter 8, "Fast Foodism Rx: Get Fresh," for more about this.)

Want proof that inverse eating reigns and has for millennia? Here's a sampling of inverse-eating wisdom in action worldwide:

- The typical Mediterranean diet—from Greece, let's say—emphasizes fruits, vegetables, grains, and legumes, with low to moderate intake of dairy foods, poultry, and fish. Small portions of red meat are eaten only occasionally, and much of the dietary fat and protein in this diet comes from fresh-pressed olive oil, feta cheese, and yogurt.
- The core of the Mexican diet is rice, beans, and corn, supplemented with meat, poultry, or fish.
- A typical meal in the Middle East is couscous, made with bulgur (cracked wheat) and bits and pieces of lamb.

- Staples of the Japanese diet are rice and tofu (made from soybeans), often supplemented with fresh fish.
- For people throughout India, whole-wheat chapati bread and lentils or legumes, greens, and other vegetables are staples. Because many Indians are Hindu and believe in *ahimsa*—causing no harm to animals—many are lactovegetarians who supplement their plant-based diet with dairy foods, especially yogurt and milk.
- National Geographic Fellow and author Dan Buettner identified regions called Blue Zones—areas across the globe with high concentrations of individuals who live to be over one hundred years old and who have low rates of heart disease, cancer, diabetes, and obesity. What each Blue Zone diet has in common is that as much as 95 percent of daily food intake comes from vegetables, fruits, grains, and legumes, while meat, dairy, sugary foods and beverages, and processed foods are avoided. (Note: Blue Zone individuals also have high levels of physical activity, low stress levels, strong social connections, and a sense of purpose.)

The takeaway: the inverse way of eating is humankind's original diet. It is the way we were—and are—meant to eat: mostly fresh, whole plant foods, with small—or no—portions of animal foods. And today's nutritional-science studies recommend this over and over. Whether your ancestry is Mediterranean, South American, African, Middle Eastern, Asian, or Indian, variations of inverse eating are your food roots.

In the next chapter, you'll discover an abundance of inverse-eating recipes from diverse cultures worldwide. But because the link between weight loss, health, healing, and Whole Person Integrative Eating is the focus of this book, here's the question both you and I need to ask: does Whole Person Integrative Eating influence weight loss?

A Food-Root Study: Inverse Eating in Action

In chapter 5, "What's a Dietary Lifestyle, Anyway? (Hint: Overeating Styles Rx)," I introduced you to Native American sculpture artist Roxanne Swentzell, who launched a gem of a WPIE-type pilot study done not too long ago with the Santa Clara Pueblo Indians in New Mexico. Swentzell's inverse-eating study provides a peek into preliminary proof that a return to one's food roots, which of course includes eating inversely and eating fresh, whole food, is the way to go for weight loss, health, and healing.

The Pueblo Food Experience is the name of Swentzell's research and education project that asked this question: what would be the health effects on Native American peoples in the U.S. who went from an over-processed, packaged, high-fat, high-sugar, lots-of-soda, chemical-laden standard American diet—if they returned to their original, ancestral diet? If they ate only original, fresh, whole food from their native area? Food from their food origins that, of course, was organic and GMO-free? A sprinkling of Native Americans of Pueblo descent (fourteen people in total) agreed to find out.

At the start of the three-month study, volunteers from six to sixty-five years old were given blood tests and weighed. A few participants were fairly healthy, but most were overweight or obese, with diabetes, heart disease, high blood pressure, liver imbalances, allergies, and more.

Here are some examples of the fresh, whole, and inverse-eating native foods enjoyed by the Santa Clara Pueblo Native Americans who followed the Native Pueblo inverse-eating diet:

- **Fruit:** wild plums, currants, strawberries, raspberries, blueberries, juniper berries, prickly-pear cactus fruits, chokecherry, serviceberry
- **Vegetables:** wild onions, wild parsley, wild spinach, watercress, mushrooms, purslane, corn, squash, tomatillos, asparagus, root vegetables, red pepper
- **Grains:** Indian rice grass, amaranth, quinoa, blue-corn masa
- **Legumes:** beans, black-eyed peas
- **Herbs and spices:** mint, rosehips, chili pods, garlic, Native salt, sumac
- **Nuts:** piñon nuts, seeds, sunflowers
- **Meat:** buffalo, deer, elk, antelope, mountain sheep
- **Poultry:** duck, geese, turkey, small birds, eggs
- **Game:** rabbits, squirrels
- **Fish:** salmon, eel

Maria Gabrielle, N.D., the naturopathic doctor who did the pre- and post-tests for the Santa Clara Pueblo Native Americans who undertook the challenge of changing their highly processed, denatured, typical standard American diets by returning to their food roots, reports these results after twelve months:

- An average weight loss of thirty-five to forty pounds; one person lost fifty pounds

- Lower cholesterol, triglyceride, blood sugar, and LDL ("bad" cholesterol) levels
- Feeling healthier and having more energy[17-20]

Says Roxanne Swentzell, who initiated The Pueblo Food Experience: "This isn't just another diet. It's more about health *within a cultural context* [italics mine] with weight being only one piece of it . . . *it's about our connection to who we were* [italics mine] . . . and choosing to continue our ancestral line."[17]

An Inverse-Eating Visit to Greece and China

Although inverse eating is atypical in America, worldwide it's the norm. Take the traditional Mediterranean diet, for instance. While many Americans interpret this as meaning white bread dipped into olive oil, white-flour pasta, and wine, it's really an example of the inverse-eating style. The traditional Mediterranean diet emphasizes a high intake of vegetables, fruits, nuts, legumes, and whole grains; a high intake of olive oil but a low intake of saturated fats; a moderately high intake of fish; occasional dairy products, meat, and poultry; and a regular but moderate intake of wine with meals.[21] In Greece, the dietary fat comes mostly from fresh-pressed olive oil (no trans fats), feta cheese (naturally low-fat), and fresh yogurt.

The Mediterranean diet caught the world's attention in the 1960s, when the World Health Organization revealed that people living in countries such as Greece, Italy, and Spain not only live longer but they also have relatively low rates of both heart disease and some cancers. Indeed, many studies have linked the Mediterranean diet to reduced risk of heart disease, cancer, and other chronic conditions. For instance, researchers at the Harvard T.H. Chan School of Public Health and its affiliate Brigham and Women's Hospital found that women who consume this diet live longer. The reference they used was longer telomeres, a biomarker linked to health and longevity.[22]

Researchers from Cornell, Oxford, and Beijing universities were so intrigued by the inverse way of eating in China that they spent a decade studying the relationship between China's ancient diet and the health of its citizens. The China Project began in 1983 when scientists began analyzing the diets of 6,500 families in 130 rural villages not yet infiltrated by Western fast food. The data they collected and began to analyze in 1990 confirmed a diet based on grains (in the South) and corn, wheat, and millet (in the North); mineral-dense vegetables; and protein from soybeans and grains. Meat and other animal-based foods were eaten only occasionally and as condiments—seemingly to improve or adjust the flavor of a dish—except during special feasts.

The researchers also discovered that the traditional, time-tested Chinese diet consisted of 75 percent calories from plant-based carbohydrates, 10 percent from protein (mostly from plant-based food), and 15 percent from fat. What a contrast to Americans' *non*-inverse way of eating: an average of 45 to 50 percent calories from mostly processed carbohydrates (white flour and sugar), 15 percent from protein (most of it from animal sources), and about 35 percent from fat.

As a matter of fact, while China was once considered to have one of the leanest populations worldwide, the influx of non-inverse American fast food is taking its toll. In 2010, out of a total population of 1.35 billion, 38.5 percent were overweight (up from 25 percent in 2002) and nearly 100 million people were obese (up from 18 million in 2005). In the United States, more than two-thirds of adults are overweight or obese. Sadly, children are catching up with the adults: for the first time in American history, children are expected to have shorter lives than their parents because of their ever-increasing weight.[23]

The takeaway: although lifestyle factors (such as physical activity, stress management, social support, and restorative sleep) in cultures may vary worldwide, inverse eating has been the perennial dietary wisdom not only for the Mediterranean and China, but also other cultures throughout the world that are healthier and thinner than Americans. The more a population deviates from its inverse-eating food origins, the more it is likely to be overweight and obese.

The Healing Secrets of Inverse Eating

What is it about the inverse way of eating that promotes weight loss, health, and healing? The answer lies in a scientific stew of jargon that was unfamiliar to most of us only a decade ago. For instance, words such as *phytochemicals* (natural "pharmacies" in plant-based food) and *antioxidants* (protective substances that keep cells healthy) now spice our food talk. And more and more, scientists are verifying the plethora of health benefits and protective power inherent in phytochemicals and antioxidants that are abundant in plant foods; not so with animal-based food, which may also contain hormones, antibiotics, and pesticides and herbicides from feed.

A sampling of phytochemicals:

- *Pectin* in strawberries may lower high cholesterol levels.
- *Phthalide* in celery may reduce high blood pressure.
- Naturally occurring substances in fruits and vegetables such as garlic, broccoli, carrots, grapes, and spinach (to name a few) may protect against cancer.

A sampling of antioxidants:

- The trace mineral *zinc* is known to boost the effectiveness of our immune system.
- Vitamins C (ascorbic acid) and E (alpha-Tocopherol) are powerful antioxidants that may lower your risk of heart disease and certain cancers.
- *Polyphenols* are the antioxidant components in green tea that have been linked to inhibiting tumor growth in animals.

David Katz, M.D., M.P.H., Director of Yale University Prevention Research Center, and one of the top nutrition researchers in the U.S.—if not the world—offers these insights into the healing nutrients of a mainly plant-based, fresh, whole-food, inverse-eating diet: "Good diets—all variations on the theme of wholesome foods, mostly plants, in sensible balanced combinations—are good in many ways. . . . They are low in added sugar, refined carbohydrates, and saturated fat. They are rich in fiber, many minerals, and vitamins—while low in sodium."[24]

Indeed, consuming lots of *fiber* found in unprocessed and unrefined fruits, vegetables, whole grains, beans and peas, and nuts and seeds, may also lower your risk of breast cancer. One type of fiber in particular, called *soluble fiber*, works its protective wonders by keeping estrogen, a natural hormone (chemical messenger), from being absorbed by your body. This is significant because high levels of estrogen have been linked with increased risk of breast cancer.

The bottom line: naturally occurring substances in plant-based foods are potentially powerful disease fighters. In the twenty-first century, we now know that along with consuming the nutrient-dense vitamins and minerals in plant-based food, consuming foods rich in fiber, phytochemicals, and antioxidants each day holds the potential to turn your refrigerator into the medicine cabinet of the future.

Implementing Inverse-Eating Wisdom

Clearly, a key theme of this chapter—indeed, this entire book—is that for most cultures worldwide, inverse eating and fresh, whole foods have been the norm for thousands of years. The more we veer away from our food roots and turn toward today's Fast Foodism overeating style, the more likely we are to overeat, to be overweight or obese, and to have diet-related chronic conditions.[11-14]

Says nutrition researcher David Katz, M.D., M.P.H., about the health and healing benefits of fresh, whole, inverse eating: "Optimal diets—any variant on the theme of wholesome, whole, mostly plant foods in sensible and time-honored combinations—are associated with longevity, vitality, and the avoidance of all chronic diseases. Because what each of us eats profoundly impacts the state and course of our health."[25] Clearly, modern nutritional science is verifying the ancient food wisdom on which our WPIE research[2,3] and inverse-eating recipes in this section are based.

Implementing inverse eating calls for blending your own ingredients for success: abundant curiosity about your personal food roots, an understanding of optimal foods (please see chapter 8, "Fast Foodism Rx: Get Fresh," for more about this), and a willingness to merge your personal mind-body health goals with ancient food wisdom and the latest science. Then you may access food's invisible power to sustain, rejuvenate, and heal—and in the process, find true nourishment.

To get you started, the next chapter, "The Recipes: Inverse Eating Around the World," takes you back to your food roots by revealing the inverse-eating meals of many ancestral diets. From ancient Mediterranean meals to authentic Native American recipes, the week of inverse-eating meals will guide you through fresh, whole, inverse-eating-based dishes for breakfast, lunch, and dinner, plus side dishes, salads, and desserts. And—from fresh, whole food, positive feelings, and mindfulness to gratitude, loving regard, and social connection—I have included *Integrative Eating Inspiration* tips for incorporating the WPIE dietary lifestyle into your fresh, whole, inverse meals.

We wish you a delightful whole person integrative—and inverse—eating journey around the world!

CHAPTER 15

THE RECIPES: INVERSE EATING
AROUND THE WORLD

The international, inverse-eating recipes in this chapter are based on the ancient-food guidelines we introduced you to in chapter 14, "Introduction to the Recipes: Fresh, Whole, Inverse." Most meals are filled with lots of fresh fruit, veggies, grains, and beans and peas, with lesser amounts of nuts and seeds and dairy, fish, poultry, or meat. If you're a vegan, you can still enjoy the recipes by choosing, for instance, nondairy milk products such as soy, almond, or rice milk—or by simply omitting dairy or other animal-based foods. The choice is yours.

Along with inverse eating, another key concept throughout the recipes—indeed, the entire book—is that of ancient food wisdom meeting modern nutritional science. With this in mind, I have modified some ancient-food ingredients in the recipes so that they include foods that have been ordained healthful by many scientific studies. A sampling: extra-virgin olive oil instead of conventional vegetable oils such as safflower or sunflower. Sausage and processed meats have been replaced with fresh, unprocessed alternatives because the World Health Organization states unequivocally that processed meats are linked with increased risk of cancer. Or if you avoid animal foods because you do not consume cholesterol-containing foods, egg whites, for instance, are an optional replacement for whole eggs.

Still . . . because Whole Person Integrative Eating is based on the ancient meaning of diet as a way of life and because it is not a restrictive way of eating, some recipes occasionally honor and include original food-root ingredients that deviate from some of today's healthful dietary recommendations. I included such foods to embrace the concept of *relaxed restraint*, a behavioral-medicine concept that supports not being rigid about what you eat.

What doesn't deviate, though, is this concept: the recipes support the Whole Person Integrative Eating guideline in chapter 8, "Fast Foodism Rx: Get Fresh," (eat fresh, whole foods in their natural state as often as possible), as well as other WPIE-based optimal-eating suggestions: go organic; select lean, grass-fed, free-range animal foods; opt for low-fat, chemical-free dairy; and choose wild fish instead of farm-raised. And please keep in mind that if organic and free range are a challenge to your budget, then choose fresh foods *as often as possible*.

Here are the cultures whose food-root cuisines you'll be visiting in this chapter:

- Tex-Mex
- Taste of Tuscany
- Mediterranean Meals
- Thai: 5 Flavors of Food
- India's Vegetarian Cuisine
- African Roots, American Soul Food
- Native American Food Roots

We wish you a taste-filled—and healthful—WPIE nutrition journey around the world.

Tex-Mex
The Original Fusion Fare

Today's Tex-Mex menu has its roots in both Texas and Mexico, each of which was part of the New Spain colony for three hundred years. This arrangement ended in the early 1800s when Mexico and Texas separated from Spain. One hundred years later, some were using the term Tex-Mex for Tejanos, people of Mexican descent living in Texas. Not too long afterward, Tex-Mex described Mexican-style cuisine of the region—especially the tasty bean, meat, and chili-pepper stew at the San Antonio Chili Stand.

Over time, combination platters of rice and beans, often topped with sour cream and melted cheese, became signature Tex-Mex fare. But it was cookbook author Diana Kennedy who, in the early 1970s, turned Tex-Mex into its own north-of-the-border regional cuisine. Today, Tex-Mex is a fusion of Mexico's ancient, traditional cuisine flavored with frontier food simmered in the spirit of Texas. Here, a day of hearty comfort food with a Tex-Mex flair.

MENU

Breakfast
Bean Chilaquiles

Lunch
Chickpea Tex-Mex Salad
Tex-Mex Chicken Chili with Black Beans
John Wilhelm's Favorite Cornbread

Dinner
Spicy Tex-Mex Salad
Sweet Potato Enchiladas
Guacamole with Chips
Arroz Con Leche (Rice Pudding)

INTEGRATIVE EATING INSPIRATION

Recipe for
Optimal Foods

When you shop for food, choose foods that are as fresh, chemical-free, and as organic as possible.

BREAKFAST

Bean Chilaquiles

Ingredients
3 corn tortillas, cut into 8 triangles each
1/2 cup salsa
1/3 cup pinto beans, cooked
1 large egg or 2 egg whites, whisked until light and blended
1/4 avocado, sliced
2 tablespoons Monterey Jack or cheddar cheese, grated
1/4 cup cilantro, coarsely chopped
Hot sauce (optional)

Directions
1. Preheat the oven to 400°F.
2. Spread the tortilla chips on a sheet and bake until crisp, about 10 minutes.
3. Spray a stainless-steel or cast-iron skillet with cooking oil. Spread the chips over a medium-high flame; stir until warm.
4. Pour the salsa over the tortillas, and cook, stirring, until the tortillas soak up most of the salsa, about 1 minute. Add the beans and stir until warm.
5. Lower the flame to medium, then push the chilaquiles to one side of the pan.
6. Crack open the egg (or use whisked egg whites), scramble it, and place it toward the center of the pan.
7. Cover the pan with a lid, and cook until the yolk or whites are done.
8. Place the chilaquiles and cooked egg or egg whites on a plate.
9. Garnish with the cheese, avocado slices, and cilantro. Sprinkle with hot sauce.

LUNCH

1. Chickpea Tex-Mex Salad

Ingredients
6 cups romaine lettuce, chopped
1 cup cherry tomatoes, halved
1 cup corn, cut fresh from cob
1/2 cup green olives, sliced
1½ cups chickpeas (optional: crisp the chickpeas in a hot skillet)
1 avocado, diced into 1/2-inch chunks
Dressing of choice

Directions
1. Toss the lettuce, tomatoes, corn, green olives, chickpeas, and avocado.
2. Gently blend the dressing with the salad materials.

2. Tex-Mex Chicken Chili with Black Beans

Ingredients
1/4 cup extra-virgin olive oil
1 pound skinless chicken breast, baked, chopped into very small pieces
1 cup black beans, cooked
1 cup onion, diced
1 teaspoon garlic, minced
1 tablespoon chili powder
2 tablespoons bouillon powder, chicken or veggie
1 cup corn, from cob
1 large jar (28 ounces) crushed tomatoes or tomato sauce
1 cup water
1/3 cup salsa

Garnishes (optional):

Shredded Mexican cheese
Cilantro
Lime wedges
Avocado slice

Directions
1. Heat oil in a large 6-quart saucepan or wok over medium heat. Do not let it smoke. Add the baked chicken pieces and stir until warmed through. Add water to pan if needed.
2. Add the beans and stir until warm.
3. Add onions, garlic, chili powder, and bouillon powder. Cook 3 to 5 minutes, until onions soften.
4. Stir in corn, tomatoes, water, and salsa. Bring to a boil, lower heat, and simmer 10 minutes.
5. Top with garnishes before serving.

3. John Wilhelm's Favorite Cornbread

Ingredients
1/2 cup butter, melted
2 eggs
1½ cups buttermilk
1½ cups coarse-ground cornmeal (white, yellow, or blue)
1 cup all-purpose flour
1/4 cup sugar
1 teaspoon baking soda
1/2 teaspoon salt
1 jalapeño, seeds removed, finely diced (optional)
1 cup corn kernels (optional)

Directions
1. Preheat oven to 375°F.
2. Over medium heat, heat a 10- or 12-inch cast-iron pan. Put 2 tablespoons of melted butter into the cast-iron pan, being sure not to let it smoke or burn.

3. In a medium bowl, combine and whisk together the remaining butter, eggs, and buttermilk—plus the jalapeño and corn kernels.

4. In a separate bowl, whisk together the cornmeal, flour, sugar, baking soda, and salt. Add the wet ingredients to the dry ingredients and blend well, but gently. Let stand for at least 10 minutes, to allow the cornmeal to absorb the liquid and "relax" to make a soft cornbread.

5. Pour the batter into the hot, buttered cast-iron pan. Place into the preheated oven and bake for 30–35 minutes. The cornbread is ready when the top is round and lightly browned. (Note: if you added 1 cup of frozen corn kernels when mixing the batter, you will need to bake the cornbread 5 minutes more.)

6. Remove from oven and let cool, about 10 minutes. Cut around the sides with a knife. Put a large plate over the top, and invert to drop the bread onto the plate. If it doesn't release immediately, recut the sides and bottom and try again. Cut into 8 pieces.

DINNER

1. Spicy Tex-Mex Salad

Ingredients
2 cups pinto beans, cooked
2 cups black beans, cooked
1/2 cup cheddar cheese, grated
1 tomato, chopped
1 bunch crisp romaine lettuce, chopped
Corn chips (baked is optimal)

Directions
1. In a large bowl, combine the pinto beans, black beans, cheese, lettuce, and tomatoes.
2. Add dressing of choice and mix well.
3. Serve with corn chips.

2. Sweet Potato Enchiladas

Ingredients
1 large sweet potato, baked with skin
1 poblano or mild chili pepper
2 large garlic cloves, minced
2 cups mushrooms, chopped
8 seven-inch corn tortillas
Enchilada chili sauce* or salsa or tomato sauce
1–1½ cups shredded Monterey Jack or cheddar cheese

Garnish:
1 scallion, diced

Directions
1. Preheat oven to 375°F.
2. Remove the stem and seeds from the chili pepper; dice into 1/4-inch pieces.
3. Spray a skillet with cooking oil. Over medium heat, sauté the pepper, mushrooms, and garlic until soft, 5–7 minutes.

4. Spray a large casserole dish with nonstick cooking oil. Mash the baked sweet potato and spread 2 tablespoons of the sweet potato and 1/4 cup mushrooms into each tortilla, then roll into a cigar shape.
5. Place the filled and rolled tortillas in the baking dish, seam side down. Fit each tortilla against each other to prevent unrolling.
6. Pour the enchilada or tomato sauce over the rolled tortillas and top with shredded cheese.
7. Bake about 25 minutes, until heated through.
8. Top with diced scallions after baking. Serve hot.

* Enchilada Chili Sauce
Add 1 eight-ounce jar salsa, 1 cup water (more if needed), 1/4 cup chopped red onion, 1/4 teaspoon oregano, 1/4 teaspoon chili powder, 1/4 teaspoon basil, 1/4 teaspoon black pepper, 1/4 teaspoon salt, 1/4 cup chopped parsley. Mix all ingredients together. Bring to a boil, reduce heat, and simmer 20 minutes.

3. Guacamole with Chips

Ingredients
1 large avocado, ripe
1/2 lime, juiced
1 tablespoon red onion, finely chopped
Salt and pepper, to taste
Corn chips, baked

Directions
1. Mash the avocado, blend in the lime juice.
2. Mix in the red onion, salt, and pepper. Add a bit of water, if necessary.
3. Serve with corn chips (baked is optimal).

4. Arroz Con Leche (Rice Pudding)

Ingredients
$1\frac{1}{2}$ cups water
1/2 cup uncooked long-grain rice

1 cinnamon stick (3 inches)
1 cup milk (cow, soy, almond, rice)
1 teaspoon vanilla extract
2 tablespoons brown sugar
3 tablespoons raisins
1 tablespoon sugar
1 teaspoon ground cinnamon

Directions

1. In a small saucepan, bring the water, rice, and cinnamon to a boil.
2. Lower heat and simmer, uncovered, 15–20 minutes or until water is absorbed.
3. Stir in milk, vanilla, brown sugar, and raisins. Bring to a boil.
4. Stirring frequently, reduce heat and simmer, uncovered, 10–15 minutes or until thick and creamy.
5. Remove cinnamon.
6. Mix together the sugar and ground cinnamon. Sprinkle over the rice pudding.
7. Let sit 15 minutes. Serve warm or cold.

Taste of Tuscany
Simple. Rustic. Fresh.

With roots reaching back to the ancient Etruscan civilization (eighth century B.C. to the third and second centuries B.C.) that predates the Roman empire, Tuscan cuisine is world-famous for its basic, high-quality meals that are full-flavored and hearty. Fish, extra-virgin olive oil, legumes, handcrafted cheese, and fresh fruit are all central to the Tuscan diet. Blend these fresh ingredients with local herbs, and the result is some of the tastiest, most mouth-watering dishes in Italy. Tuscan cooking—simple, rustic, and fresh ingredients beautifully cooked.

MENU

Breakfast
Pizza with Poached Egg
Fresh Fruit Salad

Lunch
Pappa al Pomodoro:
Tuscan Tomato-Bread Soup
Pasta with Chicken Sausage and Arugula
Polenta
Italian Salad

Dinner
Tuscan Salad
Vegetarian Lasagna
Lemon-Ricotta Granita

INTEGRATIVE EATING INSPIRATION

Recipe for
Positive Feelings

Benefit from the food-mood dance by checking in with your feelings before eating, then about 20 minutes after eating.

BREAKFAST

1. Pizza with Poached Egg

Ingredients
2 ripe tomatoes, diced
1 small scallion, finely diced
1 clove garlic, minced
2 tablespoons fresh basil, chopped
2 tablespoons Italian parsley, chopped
2 tablespoons extra-virgin olive oil
Salt and pepper, to taste
2 slices of bread (crisp crust with soft, porous texture; or multi-grain English muffin; or whole-grain artisan bread of choice)
2 slices Italian cheese, sliced very thin (such as Asiago, Gorgonzola, Parmigiano-Reggiano, pecorino pepato)
Optional:
1 large organic egg or egg whites from 2 eggs for scrambling
2 tablespoons white vinegar

Directions for Pizza
1. Preheat oven to 400°F.
2. In a medium bowl, combine tomatoes, scallion, garlic, herbs, olive oil, salt, and pepper. Sauté over medium heat until all ingredients are warm and well cooked.
3. Toast two slices of bread, then brush one side with olive oil. Line baking sheet with tinfoil. Place each slice oiled side down on baking sheet.
4. Place one slice of cheese on the toast, then press the center to create a shallow indentation for the vegetable topping. Heat until cheese is melted, 3–5 minutes. Serve warm.

Directions for Poached Egg
1. Crack 1 egg into a cup. Fill a separate, large bowl with cold water and ice. Set aside.

2. In a medium saucepan, bring 4 cups of water and 2 table-spoons white vinegar to a boil.

3. Reduce heat under the water to medium-high. Use a whisk to create a spinning whirlpool in the water, then quickly slide the egg into the swirling water. This whirlpool helps to wrap the egg white around the yolk. Cook 3–5 minutes, until desired doneness is achieved.

4. Remove egg with a slotted spoon and transfer to ice-water bath. Remove the egg with a slotted spoon.

2. Fresh Fruit Salad

Ingredients
1 cup fresh fruit, chopped (grapes, oranges, figs, peaches, pears, cherries, berries, etc.)
1 tablespoon lemon juice

Directions
Mix the fruit gently and toss with the lemon juice.

LUNCH

1. Pappa al Pomodoro: Tuscan Tomato-Bread Soup

Ingredients
1/4 cup extra-virgin olive oil
4 cloves garlic, minced
1 small yellow onion, chopped
1 red pepper, chopped
2 fresh, ripe tomatoes, chopped, or 1 jar tomatoes, chopped
2 slices of bread, toasted or stale (multigrain or artisan)
4 cups broth or hot water
Juice of 1 lime
Pinch of salt, freshly ground pepper, to taste
Fresh basil, chopped

Directions

1. Sauté the garlic and onion in olive oil until soft. Add the red pepper and tomatoes.
2. Simmer over low-medium heat for 10–15 minutes. Stir regularly and add a little warm water if needed.
3. Cut the toasted bread into large cubes and add to the tomato mixture. Mix and stir constantly until the bread is blended into the tomato sauce.
4. Add 2–3 cups of broth or hot water and stir until the bread mixture thickens into a mush. Bring to a low boil, then lower heat, cover, and simmer for 15 more minutes, adding more water if needed. Remove from heat.
5. Remove the lid, blend in the lime juice, and mix in a pinch of salt and pepper to taste.
6. When much of the broth or water has evaporated and the soup is thicker, sprinkle with the fresh basil leaves. Serve hot, at room temperature, or chilled.

2. Pasta with Chicken Sausage and Arugula

Ingredients

10 ounces pasta of choice (traditional, quinoa, corn, or buckwheat pasta, etc.)
1 tablespoon salt
2 tablespoons extra-virgin olive oil
2 small red onions, sliced into 1/2-inch wedges
Sea salt, freshly ground pepper, to taste
2 chicken sausages, cut into 1-inch slices
1 teaspoon lemon zest, finely grated
2 tablespoons lemon juice
6 cups arugula, chopped into small pieces
Parmesan cheese, finely grated

Directions

1. Preheat oven to 400°F.
2. Bring a large pot of salted water to a boil. Cook pasta until al dente. Drain.
3. In a large skillet, heat 1 tablespoon of oil over medium heat. Toss in onions, sauté, and season with salt and pepper. Cook until tender. Mix in the sausage and cook 10 more minutes.
4. Scatter the onions and small sausage pieces on a baking sheet. Roast for 25–30 minutes.
5. Combine onion, sausage, and pasta in a large bowl. Add lemon zest, lemon juice, remaining 1 tablespoon oil. Toss in arugula. Top with Parmesan. Add salt and pepper to taste.

3. Polenta

Ingredients

4 cups water
1 cup cornmeal, coarse
1 tablespoon butter, melted
1 teaspoon salt
Pepper to taste
1/2 cup ricotta (optional)

Directions

1. In a medium saucepan, bring the water to boil. Stir in the cornmeal in a slow, steady stream, stirring constantly to prevent lumps. Stir until the polenta begins to thicken (around 1 to 2 minutes). Add 1 teaspoon salt.
2. Reduce the heat so that the polenta bubbles slowly. Continue to cook, stirring occasionally, for about 20 minutes, until the polenta is thick. If it becomes too thick, stir in water to thin it a bit.
3. When the polenta is complete, turn off the heat and add the butter. Add salt and pepper to taste. Optional: stir in 1/2 cup ricotta.

4. Italian Salad

Eat like an Italian: consider having the salad after the main course to cleanse the palate and aid in digestion.

Ingredients
8 cups romaine lettuce, chopped
2 cups radicchio, chopped
2 cups cherry tomatoes, halved
1/4 red onion, thinly sliced
1/2 cup black olives, pitted and sliced
1/2 cup peperoncini or pimento peppers, chopped
2 tablespoons fresh Italian parsley, finely chopped
2 tablespoons fresh basil, finely chopped
1/2 cup shredded Parmesan cheese

Dressing:
Extra-virgin olive oil
Balsamic vinegar or wine vinegar
Salt and pepper

Directions
1. Place the lettuce and radicchio in a large bowl. Toss.
2. Toss in the remaining ingredients. Add dressing to taste.
3. Sprinkle the freshly shredded Parmesan cheese over the salad.

DINNER

1. Tuscan Salad

Ingredients
1½ cups romaine lettuce, chopped
1½ cups radicchio, chopped
1 cup baby spinach, chopped
1/2 cup provolone cheese, cut into small cubes
1/4 cup capers

Dressing:
1½ tablespoons lemon juice
1 teaspoon Dijon mustard

2 tablespoons olive oil

1/2 tablespoon capers

Directions

In a large bowl, lightly toss all salad ingredients. For dressing, combine all ingredients in a blender until smooth. Drizzle over Tuscan salad and toss.

2. Vegetarian Lasagna

Ingredients

2 large jars tomato sauce

12 large lasagna noodles, cooked

3 cups chopped, cooked spinach, water removed

2 cups ricotta cheese

4 cups mozzarella cheese, grated

1/2 cup Parmesan cheese, finely grated

1/2 cup walnuts, chopped

Directions

1. Preheat the oven to 400°F.
2. Coat a deep lasagna pan with nonstick cooking spray.
3. Cover the bottom of the pan with a layer of tomato sauce. Create a layer of pasta with 6 noodles. With 1 cup ricotta, spread large dollops on top of the noodles. Drop dollops of the spinach between the ricotta. Cover with 2 cups mozzarella.
4. Repeat all layers in the previous step.
5. Spread 2 cups of remaining tomato sauce over the grated cheese. Top with the Parmesan cheese and walnuts.
6. Cover the lasagna with tinfoil. Bake for 40 minutes. Remove from oven and let rest for 15 minutes before serving.

3. Lemon-Ricotta Granita

Ingredients

1 cup water

1/2 cup sugar

2/3 cup fresh lemon juice

1 cup ricotta cheese

2 teaspoons sugar

1 lemon, for zesting

Directions

1. In a small saucepan, stir the water and 1/2 cup sugar over high heat at a boil until the sugar dissolves. Lower heat, cover, and simmer for 5 minutes. Stir in the lemon juice. Remove mixture from heat and let it cool.

2. Pour the lemon-syrup mixture into an 8 x 8-inch square glass dish. Place it on a level surface in the freezer for 2–3 hours. Every 30 minutes, using a spatula or fork, scrape the granita away from the sides of the dish until it is completely made up of ice crystals. Tip: set a timer to remember to scrape the granita. The granita is ready when it is a light and flaky icy mixture.

3. Before serving, mix the ricotta and 2 teaspoons sugar in a medium bowl to blend. Spoon the granita into dessert bowls. Top with a dollop of the ricotta and lemon zest.

Mediterranean Meals
Ancient. Flavor-Filled. Nourishing.

For decades, the Mediterranean diet has been touted as one of the healthiest diets in the world. For good reason. Study after study has shown that the traditional Mediterranean diet lowers the risk of major chronic conditions—from heart disease and Alzheimer's to breast cancer and more—as well as overall mortality. Not surprisingly, inverse eating is the key concept of this ancient cuisine, which has been followed in European countries such as Greece, Italy, and Spain and North African and Middle Eastern countries for centuries.

The key ingredients? Fresh fruits, vegetables and tubers, whole grains and legumes, mixed nuts, and limited amounts of fish, chicken, and meat. Extra-virgin olive oil replaces butter; olives and avocado provide balanced nutrients and healthful fats; herbs and spices are used instead of salt to flavor foods; fish and poultry are enjoyed perhaps two or three times a week, while red meat is limited to no more than a few times a month. Cheese, yogurt, and Greek yogurt are typical dairy foods.

Here, a one-day cornucopia of Mediterranean dishes.

MENU

Breakfast
Lebanese Foul Moudamas (Fava Beans)
Fig Fruit Salad

Lunch
Eggplant Parmesan
Crete's Orange-Lemon Potatoes
Greek Salad (Horiatiki Salata)

Dinner
Mediterranean Salmon
Roasted Vegetables
Baked Pears

INTEGRATIVE EATING INSPIRATION

Recipe for Mindfulness Eating

Intend to be mindful.
Commit to being present.
Focus on remaining in the moment.

BREAKFAST

1. Lebanese Foul Moudamas (Fava Beans)

Ingredients
4 cups small fava beans, cooked
1 cup liquid from canned or cooked fava beans
1 teaspoon ground cumin
4 cloves garlic, minced and mashed
1/2 cup lemon juice
1/4 cup extra-virgin olive oil
1 medium red onion, finely chopped
2 ripe tomatoes, diced
1 bunch parsley leaves, finely chopped
Salt and pepper to taste

Directions
1. In a large saucepan, add the fava beans and liquid, garlic, cumin, salt, and pepper. Bring to a boil.
2. With a fork, partially mash the fava-bean mixture. Cook over medium heat for 10 minutes.
3. Stir in the lemon juice, olive oil, and half of the chopped red onion, tomatoes, and parsley. Remove from the heat.
4. Spoon the foul moudamas into a serving dish. Cover with the remaining vegetables.

2. Fig Fruit Salad

Ingredients
2 fresh figs, chopped
2 tablespoons pomegranate seeds
1 teaspoon lemon juice
2 tablespoons pistachios, coarsely ground
1/2 cup Greek yogurt

Directions
1. Toss figs and pomegranate seeds in the lemon juice.
2. Serve over the yogurt. Top with pistachios.

LUNCH

1. Eggplant Parmesan

Ingredients
2 cups tomato sauce
2 medium eggplants
2 tablespoons extra-virgin olive oil
Salt and pepper, to taste
1 cup Parmesan cheese, grated

Directions
1. Preheat oven to 325°F.
2. Trim the eggplant and cut into 1-inch rounds. Sprinkle the eggplant lightly with salt and place in a colander for 20 minutes. Rinse slices and pat dry.
3. Heat the olive oil in a frying pan and sauté the eggplant slices on both slides until they are cooked through. Add water, if needed, to keep from burning. Dry on paper towels.
4. Coat a baking dish with cooking spray. Place a layer of the eggplant slices on the bottom of the baking dish, then cover with a cup of tomato sauce and sprinkle with salt and pepper. Sprinkle with 1/2 cup Parmesan cheese. Repeat the layers until all the ingredients are used.
5. Bake at 325°F for 45–60 minutes.

2. Crete's Orange-Lemon Potatoes

Ingredients
1½ pounds potatoes, peeled and cut into quarters lengthwise
1/4 cup extra-virgin olive oil
1 cup freshly squeezed orange juice
1/2 cup freshly squeezed lemon juice
1 clove garlic, minced
2 tablespoons mustard
1/2 teaspoon dried oregano
1/2 teaspoon dried thyme
1 cup water

Sea salt and pepper, to taste

Directions
1. Preheat oven to 350°F.
2. In a large bowl, mix oil, orange juice, lemon juice, garlic, mustard, oregano, thyme, salt, pepper, and water.
3. Coat a baking pan with cooking spray.
4. Add all ingredients to the baking pan. Bake for 1 hour or until potatoes are golden brown.

3. Greek Salad (Horiatiki Salata)

Ingredients
2 tablespoons extra-virgin olive oil
2 tablespoons lemon juice
1 large garlic clove, minced
1/2 teaspoon dried oregano
1/4 teaspoon salt
1/4 teaspoon freshly ground black pepper
3 medium tomatoes, cut into wedges
1/4 red onion, sliced thinly
1/2 crisp cucumber, sliced and halved
1/2 green pepper, cut lengthwise into thin strips
4 ounces feta cheese, crumbled
10 Kalamata olives

Directions
1. Dressing: In a large jar, shake the olive oil, lemon juice, garlic, oregano, salt, and pepper.
2. In a large bowl, mix together the tomatoes, onion, cucumber, pepper, olives, and feta cheese.
3. Pour the dressing over the salad and toss gently to coat the vegetables.

DINNER

1. Mediterranean Salmon

Ingredients
4 salmon fillets, 6 ounces each
1/2 cup extra-virgin olive oil
2 teaspoons honey
1 teaspoon Dijon mustard
1 teaspoon sea salt
2 cups cherry tomatoes, halved
1/4 cup red onion, chopped
2 tablespoons green olives, pitted and sliced
2 tablespoons black olives, pitted and sliced

Directions
1. Preheat oven to 425°F.
2. Spray a large, rectangular baking pan with cooking oil. Place salmon in the pan.
3. In a small bowl, whisk together the oil, honey, mustard, and salt.
4. Spoon 1 tablespoon over each fillet.
5. In a large bowl, combine the tomatoes, onion, olives, and remaining oil mixture. Spoon over fillets.
6. Bake for 12–15 minutes, until fish flakes easily with a fork.

2. Roasted Vegetables

Ingredients
1 large potato, cut into 1½-inch chunks
12–15 small portobello mushrooms
2 red bell peppers, deseeded, cut into large chunks
1 cup red onion, coarsely sliced
1 tablespoon extra-virgin olive oil
4 garlic cloves, minced
1/2 teaspoon dried basil
1/2 teaspoon dried oregano

4 tablespoons fresh chives, chopped
1/4 teaspoon salt
1/2 teaspoon pepper, freshly ground
Juice of one lemon

Directions
1. Preheat oven to 425°F.
2. Spray a rectangular roasting dish with nonstick cooking spray.
3. In a large bowl, gently toss together the potatoes, mushrooms, bell peppers, and red onion. Distribute in roasting dish.
4. In a medium bowl, whisk together the olive oil, basil, oregano, chives, garlic, salt, and pepper.
5. Drizzle sauce over the vegetables. Toss gently to coat.
6. Roast vegetables for 45 minutes, until cooked through.
7. Top with lemon juice.

3. Baked Pears

Ingredients
2 large Bosc or Anjou pears (best for baking)
2 tablespoons brown sugar
1/2 teaspoon ground cinnamon
1 teaspoon vanilla extract
1/2 teaspoon lemon juice
5 walnut halves, finely ground
4 teaspoons orange marmalade

Directions
1. Preheat the oven to 350°F.
2. Cut pears in half lengthwise, and remove the seeds. Place pear halves on a baking sheet, cut side up.
3. Combine sugar and cinnamon and sprinkle over pears. Combine the vanilla extract and lemon juice, and drizzle on the pears.
4. Top each half with the orange marmalade and finely ground walnuts.
5. Bake 20–30 minutes, until pears are tender.

Thai: 5 Flavors of Food
A Taste-Full Cuisine

For thousands of years, ancient Eastern healing systems, such as India's Ayurveda and traditional Chinese medicine, have turned to the five flavors in food—bitter, salty, sweet, sour, and pungent—to balance meals nutritionally and enhance health. With roots back to the people who emigrated from the southern Chinese provinces into modern-day Thailand many centuries ago, early Thai cuisine had Szechwan influences, with other flavors brought by a Buddhist monk from India, by people from southern Muslim states, and later by Portuguese missionaries and Dutch traders from Europe. Today, Thai food is its own unique intermingling of the five tastes. The following recipes are a five-flavor cornucopia of dishes from throughout Thailand.

MENU

Breakfast
Thai Rice Soup (Khao Tom)
Fresh Fruit

Lunch
Tom Yum Goong (Spicy Shrimp Soup)
Thai Basil Rice (Khao Pad Horapa)
Som Tum (Green Papaya Salad)

Dinner
Miang Kham (Leaf-Wrapped Salad)
Thai Chicken with Cashews
Pad Pak Bung Fai Daeng (Morning Glory)
Banana-Lychee Dessert

INTEGRATIVE EATING INSPIRATION

Recipe for Appreciation

As you prepare food, experience heartfelt regard for the great web of life inherent in food and the act of eating.

BREAKFAST

1. Thai Rice Soup (Khao Tom)

Ingredients
8 ounces tofu, baked, cut into 1/2-inch pieces
3 cloves garlic, finely minced
1 tablespoon ginger root, grated
Small bunch cilantro stems, finely chopped
1/2 teaspoon of salt
1/2 teaspoon freshly ground black pepper
2 tablespoons fish sauce
8 cups chicken or vegetable broth
1 stalk lemon grass, smashed to release flavor
1 tablespoon ginger root, minced
4 cups brown rice, cooked
3 tablespoons soy sauce
3 tablespoons fish sauce
1/2 teaspoon pepper, ground

Garnishes:
1 scallion, finely chopped
1/4 cup fresh coriander leaves, chopped
2 red chilies, finely chopped

Directions
1. Mix the garlic, grated ginger, cilantro, salt, freshly ground pepper, and 2 tablespoons fish sauce in a large bowl. Add the baked tofu, tossing until the tofu is coated with the sauce. Set aside.
2. Bring the broth to a boil in a large pot. Add the lemon grass and tablespoon of minced ginger. Simmer for 10 minutes.
3. Add the cooked brown rice and simmer for 5 minutes. Season to taste with soy sauce, 3 tablespoons fish sauce, and 1/2 teaspoon pepper. Remove the lemon grass.
4. Add the tofu mixture to the rice soup and bring to a boil. Simmer for 5 minutes.
5. Before serving, garnish with scallion, coriander leaves, and chili.

2. Fresh Fruit

Ingredients
1 cup fruit (such as berries, apple, mango, pineapple, papaya, banana, etc.), chopped
1 tablespoon sugar
1 teaspoon dried chili flakes

Directions
1. Gently mix the fruit in a medium-size bowl.
2. Mix the sugar and chili flakes. Sprinkle mixture over the fruit.

LUNCH

1. Tom Yum Goong (Spicy Shrimp Soup)

Ingredients
1 1/2 pounds medium shrimp, deveined and cooked
8 cups water
1 bottle clam juice
1/2 cup peeled ginger, chopped
1/2 cup lemon grass stalks, peeled and chopped
1/4 cup lime juice
1/2 cup mushrooms, quartered
2 tablespoons roasted red chili paste
1 tablespoon fish sauce
2 chilies
1/4 cup green onions, chopped

Garnishes:
1/2 cup scallions, chopped
1/2 cup cilantro, chopped
6 tablespoons unsalted peanuts, chopped

Directions
1. Bring the water and clam juice to a boil in a large saucepan.
2. Add ginger, lemon grass, and lime juice; simmer 10 minutes.
3. Add mushrooms, chili paste, fish sauce, and chilies; bring to a boil.

4. Stir in shrimp, green onions, cilantro, and lime juice. Remove chilies.
5. Before serving, sprinkle with scallions, cilantro, and peanuts.

2. Thai Basil Rice (Khao Pad Horapa)

Ingredients
1 tablespoon extra-virgin olive oil
3 cloves garlic, finely chopped
1 red chili pepper, finely chopped
1/4 cup red bell pepper, sliced
1/4 cup onion slices
1/4 cup string beans, cut into 1-inch pieces
1/2 cup basil leaves
1 tablespoon soy sauce
2 cups brown rice or basmati rice, cooked
1 lime, halved

Directions
1. Heat a large skillet or wok until very hot. Add the oil, garlic, and chili. Stir-fry until garlic is golden brown.
2. Mix in the beans and red bell peppers, then the soy sauce.
3. When the beans and peppers are almost soft, add the onion slices. Stir-fry for 1 minute, until they are translucent but still firm.
4. Add the rice and mix with the other ingredients. Add the basil, then turn off the heat.
5. Squeeze the juice of the lime over the rice.

3. Som Tum (Green Papaya Salad)

Ingredients
1 large clove garlic
1/4 teaspoon salt
2 chilies, sliced
1/2 teaspoon sugar
2 tablespoons lime juice
8 cherry tomatoes, halved

1/2 pound green beans, cut into 1½-inch lengths
4–6 cups unripe green papaya, shredded
Romaine lettuce
2 tablespoons unsalted peanuts, chopped

Directions
1. Blend the garlic, salt, chilies, sugar, and lime juice in a blender until it is a paste.
2. Lightly crush the tomatoes and beans with a spoon. Place in a medium bowl and mix lightly. Add the paste and toss until the vegetables are coated with the dressing.
3. Add the shredded papaya to the vegetables and toss.
4. Line a separate, large bowl with the leaves of romaine lettuce. Add papaya salad to the bowl. Sprinkle with chopped peanuts.

DINNER

1. Miang Kham (Leaf-Wrapped Salad)

Ingredients
20 large spinach leaves or green leaves of choice
1/2 cup shredded coconut, toasted and chopped
1 large lime, cut into 1/4-inch pieces
1/4 cup scallions, cut into 1/4-inch pieces
10 small chilies, cut into 1/4-inch pieces
1/4 cup peeled ginger, cut into 1/4-inch pieces
1/4 cup dry roasted peanuts, chopped

Sauce:
1 cup thick honeycomb honey in a tub or jar of liquid honey

Directions
Arrange each of the chopped salad ingredients in small, separate bowls. Put the honey sauce in a separate bowl.

Preparation to Eat
1. Take one spinach leaf and spread a teaspoon of the honey on the leaf.

2. Put a pinch of each chopped salad ingredient on the sauce.
3. Roll the leaf, then fold the ends inward to make a packet. Eat in one bite.

2. Thai Chicken with Cashew Nuts (Gai Pad Med Mamuang)

Ingredients
Sauce:
1 tablespoon soy sauce
1 tablespoon fish sauce
1 heaping tablespoon brown sugar
1 tablespoon water

Stir-Fry:
1/2 cup cashew nuts
2 tablespoons extra-virgin olive oil
2 cloves garlic, minced
1/2 red onion, quartered
2 red chilies, deseeded and minced
8 ounces boneless, skinless chicken breast, cut into small, bite-size pieces
1 scallion, cut into 1-inch lengths

Directions
1. Whisk all sauce ingredients together in a small bowl and set aside.
2. Heat oil in a large skillet over medium-high heat. Add the cashew nuts and sauté until light brown. Set aside.
3. Over medium heat in a large skillet or wok, add the oil, garlic, onion, and red chilies. Stir-fry 3–5 minutes.
4. Add the chicken and continue to stir-fry until the chicken is cooked through.
5. Add the cashews and sauce and toss all ingredients to coat them. Remove from heat and top with the scallions.

3. Pad Pak Bung Fai Daeng (Stir-Fried Morning Glory)

Ingredients
1 bunch morning glory (also known as water spinach) or fresh greens of choice, such as Tuscan kale
1 red chili, deseeded and minced
2 cloves garlic, minced
2 tablespoons sesame oil
2 tablespoons oyster sauce
1 tablespoon brown sugar
1/4 cup vegetable stock

Directions
1. Rinse greens in cold water, then cut them into 4- to 6-inch lengths. Place on a dish towel to absorb excess water.
2. In a pestle and mortar, crush together the chilies and garlic until they are crushed but still somewhat whole.
3. Heat the oil in a wok over high heat. Add the garlic and chili, then stir-fry for about 15–20 seconds.
4. Add the greens along with the oyster sauce and sugar. Stir-fry for another 40 seconds.
5. Add the stock and sauté for 10 seconds. Remove from heat.

4. Banana-Lychee Dessert

Ingredients
1 large ripe banana
8–10 fresh and peeled, or canned and drained, lychees
1 cup coconut milk, regular or lite
1/4 cup brown sugar
Pinch of salt

Directions
1. Peel the banana, slice in half lengthwise. Cut into 2-inch pieces.
2. Over medium-high heat, pour the coconut milk into a saucepan. Stir in the sugar and salt. Mix until dissolved.
3. Add banana and lychees to the pan. Continue stirring until the bananas and lychees are warmed through (1 to 2 minutes).

India's Vegetarian Cuisine
An Ancient Tradition of Plant-Based Foods

With roots and customs dating back more than four thousand years, Hinduism is the world's oldest major religion. Today in India, almost 80 percent—about 1.2 billion people—are Hindus. Although Hindus have the reputation for being vegetarian, not all Hindus shun animal foods. Rather, vegetarianism is practiced by most Hindus in the southern regions of India and in Gujarat on the west coast.

Today, nearly 30 percent of India is vegetarian—the largest percentage of any nation. Over the centuries, India has developed a vast vegetarian cuisine, with spices providing taste and aiding digestion. The type of vegetarianism followed by millions in India is a lactovegetarian diet, meaning that they practice the inverse-eating concept of mostly plant-based fruits, vegetables, grains, legumes and pulses, and nuts and seeds, with milk products of yogurt, milk, and ghee (clarified butter) as animal-based food staples. Here, a day of this centuries-old fare.

MENU

Breakfast
Akki Roti
Tomato Thokku
Cucumber Raita

Lunch
Vegetable Sabji
Indian Lentils (Kaali Daal)
Jeera Rice

Dinner
Rajma Dal (Red-Kidney-Bean Curry)
Coriander Chutney (Dhaniye Ki Chutney)
Kachumbar Salad
Banana Sorbet
Lassi

INTEGRATIVE EATING INSPIRATION

Recipe for
Amiable Ambiance

While preparing a dish, envision how the spices you add will enhance the flavor of the food.

BREAKFAST

1. Akki Roti

Ingredients
1 cup rice flour
1/4 cup red onions, finely chopped
3 tablespoons coconut, grated
2 tablespoons carrots, shredded
1 teaspoon green chilies, finely chopped
1 teaspoon curry powder
1 teaspoon coriander leaves, finely chopped
1 teaspoon sea salt
2 cups hot water
1 teaspoon extra-virgin olive oil

Directions
1. Coat a large skillet with nonstick cooking spray.
2. In a medium bowl, mix all ingredients except water and oil. Add water slowly, to create a loose batter. Divide the dough into 3 equal parts, 1 part for each roti.
3. Heat the skillet over medium heat.
4. When the pan is hot, place a ball of batter in the center, then spread it so it's flat.
5. Puncture 8 holes in the roti. Drizzle a teaspoon of oil under, on, and inside the roti holes.
6. Cover, and cook on medium heat for 1 minute. When the roti starts to brown, flip it over to the other side and roast until golden brown. Cover with tomato thokku.

2. Tomato Thokku

Ingredients
2 large or 3 medium tomatoes
1 teaspoon ginger-garlic paste*
1 tablespoon extra-virgin olive oil
1 teaspoon mustard seeds
1/4 teaspoon turmeric powder

2 teaspoons chili powder
Salt, to taste

Directions

1. Fill a large saucepan with water, and bring the water to boil. Place the tomatoes in the boiling water, turn off heat, and cover for 10 minutes.
2. *To make the ginger-garlic paste, mince and mash 1-inch peeled ginger and 1 large garlic clove. Add 1 teaspoon extra-virgin olive oil and a pinch of salt. Continue to mash and blend.
3. After the tomatoes cool, remove the skin. Puree in a blender.
4. Oil a large skillet and heat it over medium-high heat. Add mustard seeds. When seeds split open a bit, mix in tomato puree, ginger-garlic paste, oil, turmeric powder, chili powder, and salt.
5. Cover and cook on medium flame, stirring occasionally.

3. Cucumber Raita

Ingredients

1/2 cup yogurt
1/2 cup cucumber, chopped
2 tablespoons cilantro, chopped
2 teaspoons chopped green onions
1/4 teaspoon ground coriander
1/4 teaspoon ground cumin
Sea salt, to taste

Directions

Mix all ingredients in a medium bowl. Chill, covered, until ready to serve.

LUNCH

1. Vegetable Sabji

Ingredients

2 tablespoons extra-virgin olive oil
1 teaspoon cumin seeds
1 teaspoon mustard seed
1 teaspoon coriander

1/2 teaspoon ground turmeric

1/2 teaspoon cayenne pepper

1 head cabbage, sliced and coarsely chopped

2 potatoes, coarsely chopped

1 tablespoon ginger, minced

1 tablespoon garlic, minced

1 teaspoon salt

1/4–1/2 cup water

1/4 cup fresh cilantro, coarsely chopped

Directions

1. Heat oil in a wok over medium heat. Stir in cumin and mustard seeds, and cook 1–2 minutes. Add coriander, turmeric, and cayenne; stir about 1 minute.
2. Add cabbage, potatoes, ginger, garlic, and salt; stir to coat.
3. Add enough water in the wok to steam the vegetables. Cover and cook, stirring occasionally, until potatoes and cabbage are cooked through, 30–45 minutes.
4. Remove from heat. Scatter cilantro over the vegetables.

2. Indian Lentils (Kaali Daal)

Ingredients

1 cup lentils, soaked overnight in water

3 cups water

2 large red onions, thinly sliced

2 green chilies, slit lengthwise

Salt to taste

2 tablespoons extra-virgin olive oil

2-inch piece peeled ginger, sliced

1 tablespoon garlic, minced

2 large tomatoes, cubed

2 teaspoons coriander

1 teaspoon ground cumin

1/2 teaspoon cayenne-pepper powder

1/2 cup milk (cow, soy, rice, almond)

Directions

1. In a large saucepan, bring the water to a boil. Add the soaked lentils, 1 onion, chilies, and salt to taste. Simmer until the lentils are tender. Set aside.
2. In a skillet, heat the oil and sauté the other onion until soft. Add the ginger and garlic and sauté for 1 minute. Stir in the tomatoes, coriander, cumin, and cayenne-pepper powder and sauté for 5 minutes.
3. Add the cooked lentil mixture and enough water to make the mixture thick. Simmer for 10 minutes.
4. Add the milk and mix well. Remove from heat.

3. Jeera Rice

Ingredients

1 tablespoon extra-virgin olive oil
1/2 teaspoon cumin seeds
1 cup brown basmati rice
2 cups water
1/2 teaspoon salt

Directions

1. Over medium heat, heat the oil in a medium skillet. When hot, add the cumin seeds and sauté for 1 minute.
2. Add the basmati rice, stir to coat for 2 minutes. Stir in the water and salt. When the water boils, lower heat and simmer, covered, for 15 to 20 minutes.

DINNER

1. Rajma Dal (Red-Kidney-Bean Curry)

Ingredients

2 tablespoons extra-virgin olive oil
1 teaspoon cumin seeds
2 medium red onions, finely chopped
2-inch piece peeled ginger, sliced
6 cloves garlic, minced
2 green chilies, finely chopped

2 large tomatoes, chopped into small cubes
2 teaspoons coriander powder
1 teaspoon cumin powder
1/4 teaspoon turmeric powder
2 cups red kidney beans, cooked
3 cups water
Salt to taste
Coriander leaves, chopped

Directions
1. In a large saucepan, heat the oil. Add the cumin seeds and stir until they sizzle. Add the onion and sauté until translucent.
2. Add the ginger and garlic. Sauté for 2 minutes.
3. Stir in the chilies, tomatoes, coriander, cumin, and turmeric, and sauté for 2 minutes.
4. Add the red kidney beans, water, and salt. Cook until the beans are warmed through and flavors are blended, about 10 minutes.
5. Coarsely mash about 1/2 cup of the beans, then stir. Sprinkle the coriander over the curry.

2. Coriander Chutney (Dhaniye Ki Chutney)

Ingredients
1 bunch fresh coriander leaves, coarsely chopped
8 cloves garlic
2 green chilies, deseeded, finely chopped
1/2-inch peeled ginger, finely chopped
Sea salt, to taste
2 tablespoons lemon juice
1–2 tablespoons water, if needed
1/4–1/2 cup cottage or ricotta cheese

Directions
1. Put coriander leaves in a blender; blend till leaves are crushed.
2. Add garlic, chilies, ginger, salt, and lemon. Blend till smooth. Add a little water if mixture is too thick.
3. Scoop out mixture into a bowl and mix with the cheese.

3. Kachumbar Salad

Ingredients
1/2 cup red onion, chopped
1/2 cup cherry tomatoes, halved
1/2 cup cucumber, coarsely chopped
1 small green chili, finely chopped
2 tablespoons fresh coriander, chopped
Salt, to taste
1/2 teaspoon red chili powder
1 tablespoon lemon juice

Directions
In a medium bowl, mix all the ingredients together. Adjust salt and lemon juice, to taste.

4. Banana Sorbet

Ingredients
2 ripe bananas, peeled, sliced into 1-inch pieces, and frozen
1/2 cup plain yogurt, more if needed
1 teaspoon vanilla extract
2 tablespoons almonds or pistachios, finely ground (optional)

Directions
1. Put the frozen banana pieces into a blender or food processor. Add the yogurt and blend until the batter is thick and smooth. Pulse in the vanilla extract.
2. Place servings into dessert dishes. Top with ground nuts.

5. Lassi

Ingredients
2 cups chilled fresh yogurt
1 cup chilled water
1 cup chilled milk
2 tablespoons sugar, or to taste
1 teaspoon cardamom powder
1 teaspoon rose water (optional)

Directions
Shake all ingredients in a large glass jar until frothy.

African Roots, American Soul Food

Spiced with Spirit. Stirred with Soul.
Served from the Heart.

With roots on the African continent, American soul food evolved from the sorrow of slaves on Southern plantations. Motivated by the best of what is in the human heart, the creators of African American soul food triumphed by creating a culinary art that embraces simple flavors and places a high premium on kinship, community, and friends.

Today, this true comfort food has evolved into three sub-cuisines: 1) upscale soul, which uses artisan ingredients such as heirloom vegetables and heritage meat; 2) down-home healthy, with a focus on healthful ingredients; 3) and vegan soul food, which focuses on mostly plant-based ingredients with small pieces of dried, salted, or smoked meat. Ultimately, vegan soul food is a culinary homecoming, because it's based on the original food roots of African American soul food. Here, dishes that feature typical inverse-eating soul-food meals.

MENU

Breakfast
Creamy Grits
Soul-Food Scramble

Lunch
Macaroni and Cheese
Black-Eyed Peas
Sweet Potato Unfries
Tossed Crisp Greens

Dinner
Unfried Chicken
Warmed Greens
Corn Pone
Shelly's Peach Cobbler

INTEGRATIVE EATING INSPIRATION

Recipe for
Amiable Ambiance

When you eat, choose pleasant surroundings and discern whether you—and people around you—have positive emotions.

BREAKFAST

1. Creamy Grits

Ingredients
4 cups water
3/4 teaspoon salt
1 cup yellow or white grits
1 cup milk of choice (cow, soy, rice, almond)
1/4 teaspoon black pepper
1 tablespoon butter, unsalted

Directions
1. In a medium saucepan, bring water and salt to a boil. Add grits gradually, stirring constantly with a wooden spoon.
2. Reduce heat so grits are at a low simmer, covered. Stir frequently until water is absorbed, about 15 minutes.
3. Stir in the milk and simmer, partially covered. Stir occasionally to keep grits from sticking to bottom of pan, until liquid is absorbed and grits are thick.
4. Stir in pepper and butter until melted.

2. Soul-Food Scramble

Ingredients
2 cloves garlic, minced
2 cups collard greens, chopped
2 ripe tomatoes, chopped
4 large eggs or 8 egg whites
1/4 teaspoon salt
1/4 teaspoon black pepper, freshly ground
1/4 cup sharp cheddar cheese, shredded

Directions
1. Coat a large skillet with nonstick cooking spray.
2. Add garlic and sauté 2 minutes. Add water if needed to keep the garlic from sticking.

3. Mix in the collard greens and tomatoes. Sauté until soft. Spray the pan with cooking spray, or add water if veggies begin to stick.

4. In a bowl, whisk together eggs or egg whites, salt, and pepper.

5. On low-medium heat, add mixture to skillet; cook without stirring until eggs begin to set on bottom. Stir egg mixture gently after eggs start to set on bottom. Sprinkle with cheese, cover, and cook until eggs are firm and cheese is melted.

LUNCH

1. Macaroni and Cheese

Ingredients
3 cups elbow macaroni, uncooked
2 teaspoons sea salt
4 cups sharp cheddar cheese, shredded
2 cups Monterey Jack cheese, shredded
1½ cups milk
2 cups half-and-half
3 eggs
1 teaspoon salt
1/2 teaspoon freshly ground black pepper

Directions
1. Preheat oven to 350°F.

2. In a large pot, bring 6 cups of water with 2 teaspoons of salt to a boil. Add macaroni, cook until firm, drain, rinse in cold water, and set aside.

3. In a large bowl beat the eggs. Whisk in the milk, then the half-and-half.

4. Add and mix in 3 cups of the cheddar and 1½ cups of the Monterey Jack cheeses. Fold in the pasta, salt, and black pepper.

5. Coat a 9x9 inch baking dish with nonstick spray. Pour the macaroni mixture into the baking dish. Top the macaroni by sprinkling it with the remaining cheeses.

6. Bake uncovered for 35–45 minutes. Do not overbake. Let cool for 10 minutes until fully set.

2. Black-Eyed Peas

Ingredients
2 tablespoons extra-virgin olive oil
3 cups yellow onion, finely chopped
4 cloves garlic, finely chopped
2 cups vegetable stock
4 cups black-eyed peas, dry
5 cups water
2 fifteen-ounce jars of whole tomatoes
3 tablespoons tomato paste
2 tablespoons brown sugar
Salt and pepper, to taste

Directions
1. Soak the black-eyed peas in water overnight.
2. In a large pot, heat the oil over high heat. Add the onions and garlic, and cook until onions are translucent. Add the vegetable stock, black-eyed peas, water, tomatoes, tomato paste, and brown sugar, and bring to a boil.
3. Lower heat and simmer until peas are tender. Add salt and pepper.

3. Sweet Potato Unfries

Ingredients
2 sweet potatoes, cut 3–4 inches long, 1/4 inch wide
1/3 cup extra-virgin olive oil
1/3 cup cornstarch
1 teaspoon garlic powder
1 teaspoon smoked paprika
1 teaspoon black pepper
Sea salt, to taste

Directions
1. Preheat oven to 425°F.
2. Toss the unfries in olive oil until lightly coated.

3. Whisk together the cornstarch, garlic powder, paprika, and black pepper. Coat the unfries with the mixture.
4. Spray a baking sheet with cooking spray. Arrange potatoes in a single layer on the baking sheet.
5. Bake until crispy, 45–60 minutes. Remove the pan from the oven, transfer it to a cooling rack. Season the unfries by coating them with salt, to taste.

4. Tossed Crisp Greens

Ingredients
2 cups romaine lettuce, coarsely chopped and chilled
1/4 cup freshly grated Parmesan cheese
1 tablespoon extra-virgin olive oil
2 teaspoons balsamic vinegar

Directions
Toss the Parmesan cheese with the lettuce. Add the olive oil and balsamic vinegar. Toss gently.

DINNER

1. Unfried Chicken

Ingredients
2 cups buttermilk
1 tablespoon hot pepper sauce
2 chicken-breast halves
2 chicken legs
2 chicken thighs
1½ cups multigrain breadcrumbs
1 cup panko breadcrumbs
3 tablespoons Parmesan cheese, finely ground
2 teaspoons garlic powder
1 teaspoon black pepper, ground
1 teaspoon cayenne pepper
1 teaspoon smoked paprika
1 teaspoon sea salt

Directions

1. Preheat oven to 400°F.
2. In a large bowl, mix buttermilk and hot sauce, then add chicken. Toss chicken to coat it. Marinate in refrigerator for at least 1 hour.
3. Coat a baking sheet with cooking spray.
4. In a large bowl, mix breadcrumbs, Parmesan cheese, garlic powder, black pepper, cayenne pepper, smoked paprika, and salt.
5. Remove the bowl with the chicken from the refrigerator. Take each piece of chicken, shake off excess marinade, and coat each piece with the breadcrumb mixture. Arrange breaded chicken on the baking sheet.
6. Refrigerate breaded chicken for 30 minutes.
7. Before baking, lightly coat chicken pieces with cooking spray. Bake until chicken starts to brown, 15–20 minutes. Turn pieces and bake another 15–20 minutes, until the chicken is cooked and the coating is crisp.

2. Warmed Greens

Ingredients

2 tablespoons extra-virgin olive oil
10 cups chard, coarsely chopped
6 beet-green stems, cut into 1-inch pieces
1 medium red onion, coarsely chopped
2 scallions, cut into 1-inch pieces
6 cloves garlic, minced
1/2 small jalapeño pepper, minced
Salt and pepper, to taste

Directions

1. In a large skillet or wok, add the olive oil. Over medium-high heat (not smoking), sauté the onions until translucent, then add the scallions. Lower heat to low-medium, and add the garlic and jalapeño pepper; stir for 3 minutes.
2. Return heat to medium-high, then stir in the chard and beet stems. Add 1/4 cup water. Continue stirring gently until the

greens are soft. Add salt and pepper.

3. On low heat, place a lid on the pan and let steam for 7 minutes. Turn off heat.

3. Corn Pone

Ingredients
2 tablespoons butter, melted
2 cups yellow cornmeal, finely ground
1/2 teaspoon salt
1½ cups cold water (or enough to make the batter similar to pancake batter)
1 teaspoon baking powder
1/2 cup milk

Directions
1. Preheat oven to 475°F.
2. Coat a 9- or 10-inch iron skillet with the butter and place it in the oven.
3. Mix the cornmeal, salt, baking powder, milk, and water so that the batter is slightly thick, but thin enough to pour.
4. With oven mitts, remove the hot skillet from the oven and pour in the batter, making 3- or 4-inch rounds.
5. Bake for 15 minutes or until golden brown. Turn up the heat to broil, if needed, to make the corn pone golden and crispy.

4. Shelly's Peach Cobbler

Ingredients
Fruit:
3–4 cups ripe peaches, sliced
1½ cups water
1 teaspoon cinnamon
1½ cups sugar
1/4 cup cold water
3 tablespoons cornstarch

Batter:

1 tablespoon baking powder

1 cup flour

1 cup sugar

1 teaspoon salt

4 tablespoons butter (melted)

1 teaspoon vanilla extract

Topping:

2 tablespoons sugar

1 teaspoon cinnamon

1 tablespoon unsalted butter

Directions

Fruit:

1. Mix fruit, water, cinnamon, and sugar in saucepan, then boil until thickened slightly.
2. Lower heat to gentle simmer. While fruit mixture is warming, mix 1/4 cup cold water with 3 tablespoons cornstarch. After the fruit has boiled and thickened, stir the cornstarch mixture into the fruit mixture to thicken it as it boils. Keep stirring while thickening to prevent lumps.

Batter:

3. Coat a 9 x 13-inch casserole dish with nonstick cooking spray.
4. Mix baking powder, flour, sugar, and salt. Add the butter and vanilla extract. Pour into casserole dish. Add prepared fruit. Do not stir.

Topping:

5. Mix together the sugar and cinnamon. Sprinkle across top. Dot with butter.
6. Bake in pre-heated 350°F oven until golden brown.

Native American Food Roots
A Return to Indigenous Ingredients

When Native American sculptress Roxanne Swentzell and thirteen other members of the Santa Clara Pueblo—a Native American tribe in New Mexico—returned to the foods their ancestors ate, their health flourished. I told you about their healing-food odyssey in chapter 5, "What's a Dietary Lifestyle, Anyway? (Hint: Overeating Styles Rx)." From obesity and heart disease to diabetes and depression, many of the conditions that plagued Roxanne and her indigenous community reversed—and simply stopped—when they returned to their food roots.

Here, a taste of the original Native American cuisine from the region of Roxanne's ancestors—the Tewas of New Mexico. These are the original foods of the Pueblo peoples, which restored the health of Roxanne and her indigenous family and friends. Recipes are from Roxanne's The Pueblo Food Experience Cookbook.

MENU

Breakfast
Corn Tortillas
Wild-Spinach Tomatillo Omelet
Berry-Veggie Smoothie

Lunch
Butternut-Squash Soup
Piñon Trout
Dandelion Greens

Dinner
Santa Clara Bean Loaf
Baked Squash
Three-Sister Salad
Grandma Marian's Cookies

INTEGRATIVE EATING INSPIRATION

Recipe for
Amiable Ambiance

Reclaim your Social
Nutrition heritage.
Consider how you
can set a social table
with family, friends,
or coworkers.

BREAKFAST

1. Corn Tortillas

Ingredients
2 cups cornmeal
1½ cups warm water
1/8 teaspoon salt

Directions
1. Mix all ingredients together until dough is no longer sticky.
2. Form the dough into balls and flatten them by hand or with a tortilla press.
3. Cook the flattened dough on a griddle until brown. Turn and repeat on the other side.

2. Wild-Spinach Tomatillo Omelet

Ingredients
1 large tomatillo
1/2 cup wild spinach
2 turkey eggs
Salt

Directions
1. Chop tomatillo into small slices. Chop spinach into small slices.
2. Beat turkey eggs and add all ingredients together.
3. Cook in a saucepan and stir constantly until done. Add salt to taste.

3. Berry-Veggie Smoothie

Ingredients
5 organic strawberries
4 stems raw organic asparagus
Handful of blueberries
3 pitted prunes
1 cup water

Directions
1. Place all fruits and vegetables into a blender.
2. If you would like, add ice. Blend thoroughly.

LUNCH

1. Butternut-Squash Soup

Ingredients
1 butternut squash
Water
3 cups turkey broth
Salt (to taste)

Directions
1. Cut squash into halves or quarters. Clean seeds out of squash. Place in a baking dish with about 1 inch of water.
2. Bake squash at 375°F for 1 hour. When squash is soft, place it in a blender. Add turkey broth until it covers the pieces of squash in the blender. Blend thoroughly.
3. Pour the mixture into a stockpot and simmer for 1 hour. When it is done, add salt as needed.

2. Piñon Trout

Ingredients
1/8 cup piñon nuts, shelled
1/8 teaspoon salt
1 trout

Directions
1. Smash piñons into crumbs. Add salt.
2. Rub piñon/salt crumb mixture all around the trout. Leave any excess mixture on top of the trout.
3. Cook in oven at 350°F until done, about 20 to 30 minutes.

3. Dandelion Greens

Ingredients
Wild dandelion greens (as many as you would like to eat)

Wild dandelion greens must be gathered in early spring. Once they flower, the leaves taste bitter, but the flowers can still be eaten whole.

Directions
Eat greens fresh in a salad in early spring or boil greens to create a warm vegetable side dish.

DINNER

1. Santa Clara Bean Loaf

Ingredients
1/2 onion
1 large tomatillo
4 cups cooked mashed beans
1/2 cup crumbly corn masa
1/2 cup sunflower seeds
1 turkey egg
1 teaspoon salt

Directions
1. Mince onion thoroughly. Chop tomatillo into cubes.
2. Mix all ingredients together. Once they are thoroughly mixed, pack them into a loaf pan.
3. Bake at 350°F for 45 minutes.

2. Baked Squash

Ingredients
1 winter squash
1/8 teaspoon salt
Currants and shelled piñon nuts (optional)

Directions
1. Cut squash in halves. Scrape out seeds and pulp. (Save seeds. These can be roasted and eaten as snacks or used as a base for oil.)

2. Salt squash halves and place in the oven. Bake in oven at 350°F until squash is soft (about 1 hour).
3. To add flavor, add currants and piñon nuts before baking squash. Salt to taste.

3. Three-Sister Salad

Ingredients
1/2 cup white corn from 2 cobs
1/4 cup prickly pear pads
1/2 cup yellow squash
1/2 cup black beans
1/2 cup squawbush berry water*
Salt

Directions
1. Boil corn until tender. Let corn cool before removing kernels from the cob. Place kernels in a large mixing bowl.
2. Rinse prepared (thorns removed) prickly pear pads. Dice them into cubes. Dice squash into cubes as well. Place squash and prickly pear pads into a hot frying pan and lightly sauté them. Once they are sautéed, add them to the mixing bowl with the corn.
3. Cook the black beans. Put beans, corn, squash, and prickly pear pads into the large mixing bowl. Add squawbush berry water. Salt as needed.

*Place ripe berries in water, shake them, and drain out the water.

4. Grandma Marian's Cookies

Ingredients
1/2 cup cacao powder or niblets
1½ cups water
1/2 cup currants or dried strawberries
1 cup cornmeal flour (white, blue, or yellow)
1 cup piñon nuts, shelled (or pumpkin or sunflower seeds)

Directions

1. Preheat oven to 350°F.
2. Boil cacao powder or niblets in water. After boiling, strain out the cacao.
3. Place currants or strawberries in the liquid and boil lightly until they have softened.
4. Mix together cornmeal flour and nuts or seeds. Add this to the cacao liquid mixture. The consistency should be like that of cookie dough.
5. Place spoonfuls of the mixture onto a baking sheet. Bake for 30 minutes.

Note: If an ingredient is unusual or hard to find—such as turkey eggs—please use an easier-to-find alternative that's as close as possible to the original, such as an organic, free-range, grass-fed chicken egg. Or replace a tomatillo with a heritage tomato. Or wild dandelion greens with fresh dark greens, such as kale or spinach.

Recipes reprinted with permission of the publisher from *The Pueblo Food Experience Cookbook: Whole Food of Our Ancestors* edited by Roxanne Swentzell and Patricia M. Perea (Museum of New Mexico Press, 2016).

OUR THOUGHTS ON RESHAPING THE OBESITY CRISIS IN AMERICA

By identifying the interrelated web of what (food choices), how (eating behaviors), and why (Emotional Eating) we overeat and gain weight, our research on Whole Person Integrative Eating (WPIE) expands our understanding about the underlying, multimodal, whole-person causes of overeating, overweight, and obesity. In this epilogue, Larry and I are sharing our thoughts about how our Whole Person Integrative Eating model and program may be integrated into communities throughout the U.S.—and in this way, contribute to turning the tide of the escalating obesity epidemic.

During presentations, I often offer the following scenario for consideration.

Imagine it's wintertime at 6:30 p.m. and you're in your car, driving home from work. It's dark and cold outside, you're fairly hungry (if one is famished and ten is stuffed, you're at, say, level three), and you won't be home for half an hour. As you drive in the rush-hour traffic, you think about the meal that awaits you. You know that your grandmother—who lives with you, your spouse, and your three adolescent children—has been preparing a traditional Italian dinner for the past few hours. You know that when you enter your home, your first greeting will be the aroma of her freshly made meal.

As you hang up your coat, you'll glance at the dining table, set as always for six. Sighing with delight, you'll think about how welcoming it looks and how lucky you are to come home to a home-cooked meal with your family.

When I ask people to share their reaction to this scene, I often hear sighs of satisfaction and comments such as "I feel peaceful." Fresh food. A homemade meal. Family dinners. A warm, welcoming atmosphere. Understanding that optimal eating is more than the food you eat. Bringing an attitude of gratitude to meals, savoring and "flavoring" food with loving regard, and enjoying food with others. In other words, this scene is about eating with awareness of the Whole Person Integrative Eating dietary lifestyle.[1] It is having a dining experience that is the opposite of the new-normal overeating styles we have been telling you about in this book that lead to overeating, overweight, and obesity: a diet of mostly fast, processed food, eaten alone while filled with negative emotions or while doing other activities or on the run; it is the opposite of dieting and not really tasting and enjoying your food.[2,3]

Is it realistic to ask people to make such profound Whole Person Integrative Eating changes in both their food choices and eating behaviors? One country thinks so: Canada. In January 2019, the new Canada's Food Guide broke precedent with its earlier, decades-old, more traditional dietary guidelines, and instead it praised and encouraged a way of eating that tells Canadians not only *what* to eat for health and healing (mostly fresh, whole food), but also *how* to eat: with mindfulness, cooking at home more often, eating meals with others, and enjoying food.[4,5] Canada's key message: "Eat well today and every day."[6]

In other words, Canada is espousing food and eating guidelines that complement and support the Whole Person Integrative Eating re-visioning of nutritional health:[7] our dietary-lifestyle approach to food and eating that is more in tune with the time of Greek physician Hippocrates (460–370 BC) and the wisdom traditions, when *diet* meant "way of life" rather than today's definition as a "restrictive, regimented, prescribed way of eating." At its core, Canada is championing a relationship to food and eating that, our research on WPIE has shown, can help people achieve not only optimal weight and physical health but also emotional, spiritual, and social well-being.[1-3]

In this epilogue, we'd like to share our thoughts about how the Whole Person Integrative Eating dietary lifestyle might serve as a comprehensive, ancient-new way of eating that could be taught—experientially—and integrated into communities throughout the U.S. and, in this way, address America's obesity crisis.

Whole Person Integrative Eating Research . . . So Far

Here's where the research on Whole Person Integrative Eating stands as of this writing:

- We have conducted a large cross-sectional study that led to 1) discovery of the overeating styles 2) and validating the new-normal overeating styles as accurate, stable predictors of overeating. What is so very exciting about our research from this national study is that each eating style is related to overeating and most to obesity, and together the seven overeating styles account for over half the variance in overeating.[2]

- When researcher Erica Oberg, N.D., M.P.H., applied the overeating styles and the Whole Person Integrative Eating intervention to people with type 2 diabetes, she found that reducing overeating *behaviors* (Emotional Eating, Food Fretting, Sensory Disregard, Task Snacking, Unappetizing Atmosphere, and Solo Dining) was a stronger predictor of lowering A1C (blood-glucose) levels than *what* (Fast foodism) research participants ate.[8,9]

- Our research on Whole Person Integrative Eating with health-psychology students at San Francisco State University revealed that two one-hour lectures—in addition to filling out our "What's Your Overeating Style? Self-Assessment Quiz"[10] before and after the lectures—were enough to help students improve on each of the overeating styles. Indeed, the students' overall changes in their food choices (what they ate) and eating behaviors (how they ate) were significant (meaning not by chance) but moderate, and they were all in the same positive direction.[11]

- When researcher Erin Yaseen replicated our discovery about the link between the overeating styles, overeating, and being overweight,[1,2] she found that those who overate and were obese scored especially high in the Fast Foodism and Sensory Disregard overeating styles, while those who followed the elements of our Whole Person Integrative Eating dietary lifestyle overate less and had a lower percentage of body fat. Yaseen concluded that "Integrative eating may improve our understanding of behavioral contributors to obesity."[12]

We believe these research findings suggest that WPIE has the potential to provide people with the self-care insights and specific whole-person dietary lifestyle skills they need to improve what and how they eat and in turn improve their weight and well-being. Because of this, we have arrived at a radically different understanding—from the perspective of conventional weight-loss strategies—of what it takes to attain and maintain weight loss. We believe it calls for a multidimensional WPIE approach: one that includes nutrient-dense, fresh, whole foods (Biological Nutrition); positive emotions while eating (Psychological Nutrition); sensory, appreciative, mindful regard (Spiritual Nutrition); and dining with others in a pleasant atmosphere (Social Nutrition).

First Steps

Surely, transforming today's new-normal overeating styles into a WPIE dietary lifestyle—a new way of eating and living, if you will—is no easy task. The first step would be to *show*—not tell—people how to eat optimally in a randomized, controlled clinical trial with a to-be-defined community population. This WPIE research project would be designed to demonstrate that the Whole Person Integrative Eating dietary lifestyle is indeed a viable intervention for addressing overeating, overweight, and obesity. Once this is accomplished, the WPIE model and program could be applied on a national level.

For the benefits to last a lifetime, practice, practice, practice needs to accompany the training. Because of this, we are suggesting that the nationwide Whole Person Integrative Eating dietary-lifestyle intervention would be *implemented over a generation.* We think this is what is necessary to create a cultural shift, as with, for instance, the shift that occurred away from smoking over decades.

Here are our thoughts about how a WPIE dietary-lifestyle intervention might look.

Vision for a WPIE Dietary-Lifestyle Intervention

To address the number-one public-health problem in the U.S.—the ever-escalating numbers of overweight and obese children, adolescents, and adults—we are proposing an innovative, integrative, sustainable, whole-family, and community-centered Whole Person Integrative Eating program, *intended to be implemented over a generation.* To accomplish this, we are proposing a clinical trial designed to prevent and turn the tide of the growing number of overweight and obese children, adolescents, and adults in the U.S.A. by creating an ongoing, comprehensive, culturally sensitive, community-based Whole Person Integrative Eating program . . . again . . . *over twenty years*.

The population. Coaching would be a key ingredient throughout the community-based model for individuals, families, and communities throughout the United States. In each get-together, participants would learn—through personal, hands-on experience—how to replace the new-normal overeating styles we have identified (see chapter 2, "Meet the Overeating Styles 'Family': 7 Root Causes of Overeating," for more about this)[2] with the time-tested, scientifically sound, biological, psychological, spiritual, and social nutrition ingredients of Whole Person Integrative Eating: fresh, whole foods; positive emotions; mindfulness; gratitude; loving regard; and dining with others in a pleasant emotional atmosphere and physical environment.

This would mean teaching selected participants how to practice the WPIE dietary lifestyle as a way of eating (and living) that nourishes multidimensionally. At the same time, participants would be given the insights and skills they need to replace the new-normal overeating styles with a way of eating that enhances physical, emotional, spiritual, and social well-being each time they eat.[1,2]

To accomplish this, we are suggesting training and treating individuals, siblings, parents, grandparents, and nannies who are either in the ninety-fifth percentile for height and weight or simply interested in learning a scientifically sound optimal-eating program—with an intensive Whole Person Integrative Eating dietary-lifestyle intervention.

The WPIE program. Participants in the WPIE dietary-lifestyle intervention would meet twice weekly in a faith center (such as the local church), a community center (such as the local YMCA), an office conference room, or a school or university. At each meeting, participants would bring potluck dishes based on WPIE guidelines; individuals or the entire group would take a thirty-minute walk before eating; then they would meet at the Center to enjoy a meal together; afterward, they would discuss successes and challenges.

During the get-together, individuals would learn the elements of Whole Person Integrative Eating based on a curriculum that includes WPIE education and counseling, cooking classes and community-created cookbooks; and support services. After a shared meal, each meeting would wrap up with a group session designed to discuss successes and obstacles and how challenges may be overcome.

Cultural sensitivity. To honor the key concept of ancient food wisdom, on which the Whole Person Integrative Eating model and program is based,[7,13] the what-to-eat WPIE guideline would focus on consuming mostly fresh, whole, plant-based foods (fruits, veggies, whole grains, legumes, nuts and seeds) with lesser amounts of lean and low-fat dairy, fish, poultry, and meat; what we call *inverse eating* (see chapter 14, "Introduction to the Recipes: Fresh, Whole, Inverse," for more about this).

At the same time, we are suggesting that the what-to-eat WPIE guideline—*eat fresh, whole foods in their natural state as often as possible*—be applied to and adapted by individual cultures throughout the U.S. For instance, Hispanics of, say, Mexican heritage might choose a traditional inverse Mexican meal of rice and beans with chili relleno (either a veggie or chicken version); African Americans may opt for a Sunday church meal of sautéed greens and *un*fried chicken; and people from India may choose to follow the lactovegetarian diet (plant-based foods supplemented with dairy) of many Hindus. In this way, instead of an "expert" *telling* people what to eat, individuals may turn the fresh-whole-food guideline into a fulfilling, culturally sensitive eating experience based on their personal food roots.

Community support. When individuals or family members meet twice weekly, program participants will learn optimal WPIE-based eating and dietary-lifestyle skills that will be supported and sponsored by community groups (e.g., local spiritual and religious organizations, schools, Whole Foods Market or other health-food stores, local supermarkets, community centers, the YMCA, local medical centers, worksites, the local Women, Infants, and Children nutrition-education program, Trips for Kids (safe bike and walking paths), etc.); and individuals such as physicians, psychologists, allied-health practitioners, and more.

Long-term sustainability. To reap the rewards, the WPIE dietary-lifestyle intervention is designed to be practiced throughout one's lifetime. While we recognize that an intensive program of dietary-change instruction and practice is resource intensive and that continued funding will be needed to maintain its administration, every effort will be made to have the community support the project.

To ensure sustainability, participating individuals and families in the first year of the WPIE dietary intervention would be selected based on their ability and willingness to be trained to become teachers and leaders of the program in the community; in this way, they would become a key resource. Such a structure would reduce teaching costs in ensuing years, while at the same time it would enable participants to serve and reach a larger group of individuals and families.

Teachers teaching teachers. We envision the ideal implementation of the WPIE dietary-lifestyle intervention as occurring over a generation because we think this is what it will take for people to become familiar with and internalize the Whole Person Integrative Eating dietary lifestyle. To expedite this, we suggest that trained program participants teach WPIE principles to succeeding groups. In this way, individuals, children, and their families will have ongoing access to optimal (and anti-weight-gain) eating practices; at the same time, they will be empowered both to live in and to continue to create a safe community that supports an optimal and healthful dietary lifestyle.

WPIE: A Re-Visioning of Nutritional Health

"[Whole Person Integrative Eating] provides a fresh perspective on our epidemic of overeating, overweight, and obesity. [It] identifies underlying causes of overeating and ensuing weight gain that, if replicated, could signal a paradigm shift in the field of nutrition," wrote David Riley, M.D., about our Whole Person Integrative Eating research findings.[14] We agree. This is because, ultimately, the Whole Person Integrative Eating dietary lifestyle we're proposing as a community and nationwide intervention is a re-visioning of nutritional health.

Our findings also propose this question: could returning to our food roots—going back to a dietary lifestyle that nourished humankind physically, emotionally, spiritually, and socially for millennia—be the answer to turning the tide of today's pandemic of overweight, obesity, and other diet-related chronic conditions? Our research suggests this is so,[1,2] as does Canada's breakthrough 2019 dietary guidelines for its citizens.[4-6] Clearly, evaluation with other populations is the next step.

We know. We're proposing quite an ideal vision: to help the millions of overweight and obese Americans who eat based on the new-normal overeating styles, we envision engaging people throughout the U.S. in a comprehensive, experiential *new* new-normal, *whole-systems* research project,[15] meaning our Whole Person Integrative Eating model and program. And we are proposing that our WPIE intervention take place *over a generation* so that Americans of all ages learn a new normal way of relating to food and eating.

To accomplish this, the Whole Person Integrative Eating dietary lifestyle would join with the many other quality organizations working to combat the obesity pandemic throughout the United States. Together, we would address the complexity of creating a new-normal relationship to food and eating that could lead to overcoming overeating, overweight, and obesity—and in the process, reshape the obesity crisis in America.

THE EVOLUTION AND SCIENCE BEHIND THE OVEREATING STYLES

By Larry Scherwitz, Ph.D.

This appendix is a summary of the origins and development of the concept of eating styles and their relationship to overeating, overweight, and obesity. It begins with Deborah's and my discovery of ancient-food-wisdom guidelines, proceeds to our discernment of consistencies in these guidelines, develops and validates measures of these consistencies, and finally, shows that *not* following Whole Person Integrative Eating guidelines is consistently related with overeating, overweight, and obesity.

Ancient food wisdom. Through food-related research into the world's wisdom traditions, cultural traditions, Eastern healing systems, and Western nutritional science (discussed in chapter 1, "Discovering Whole Person Integrative Eating"), Deborah identified the many ways in which cultures regarded, experienced, prepared, and shared food for millennia—prior to the evolution of nutritional science in the twentieth century. Findings from this research were published in Deborah's first book, *Feeding the Body, Nourishing the Soul*.[1]

To make sense of the large amount of food wisdom, when we looked for consistencies, we found six perennial principles, which evolved into the Whole Person Integrative Eating (WPIE) program: 1) eat fresh, whole food in its natural state as often as possible; 2) be aware of feelings and thoughts before, during, and after eating; 3) bring moment-to-moment nonjudgmental awareness to each aspect of the meal; 4) appreciate food and its origins from the heart; 5) savor and "flavor" food with loving regard; (6) and unite with others through food. Each theme is discussed in detail in Deborah's book *The Healing Secrets of Food*.[2]

Deborah also created the seventy-six-item questionnaire we now call "What's Your Overeating Style? Self-Assessment Quiz,"[3] which includes sets of questions designed to evaluate each of these six perennial themes. Each question asks about the frequency of practicing various food choices and eating behaviors on a six-point scale ranging from *never* to *always*. The original questionnaire, which contained eighty questions, was the questionnaire used in the original research reported in *Explore: The Journal of Science and Healing*. The revised seventy-six-item "What's Your Overeating Style? Self-Assessment Quiz" used in this book is our updated, modified version of the questionnaire. The seventy-six-item questionnaire is the version we refer to throughout *Whole Person Integrative Eating*.

Research design. We were able to validate the questionnaire when the editor at *Spirituality & Health* magazine[4] invited Deborah to write a feature article about Whole Person Integrative Eating and to create an e-course on her Whole Person Integrative Eating model and program.[5] To take the course, participants were required to fill out the quiz both prior to and after completing the six-week, eighteen-lesson e-course.

The research design is a cross-sectional study of a national sample of 5,256 readers of *Spirituality & Health* who took the online WPIE course. We also obtained data from 192 people who completed the eighty-item questionnaire after taking the six-week e-course.[6] We used the quiz to measure how often people in the study practiced the six perennial themes we had identified; and data on height, weight, and demographics provided additional information.

Because it provided insights into what evolved into the overeating styles, a critical question included in the questionnaire asked about the frequency of overeating. To assess whether the remaining seventy-nine questions were related to the frequency of overeating, I computed bivariate correlations between these questions and their reported overeating frequency. I found that seventy-eight of the seventy-nine questions were significantly correlated with overeating in the predicted direction. All negative items correlated with more frequent overeating, and positive items correlated with less frequent overeating.

Conceptual validation of the overeating styles. Because there were too many correlations to discuss separately, I used an analytic technique called factor analysis to determine whether the seventy-nine items in the questionnaire would cohere into a manageable number of patterns of food-related practices. Because the sample size was large (5,256), I used all seventy-nine items in one analysis. The factor analysis showed a strong intercorrelation of items into seven separate groups.[6] In this way, they validated the six perennial elements as eating styles or daily practices in a contemporary population.

As interesting, the Varimax rotation helped me identify the elements that are independent of one other. For example, items measuring "heartfelt regard for food" are separate from items measuring "mindfulness" or "social atmosphere" while eating. This means that each overeating style deserves separate attention in both evaluation and making changes in food choices and eating behaviors to improve one's relationship to food.

Assessing reliability. The first step to assess the reliability of the overeating styles was to 1) randomize the 5,256 sample into two equally sized groups 2) and repeat the factor analysis. The results, which showed an almost exact overlay of factors, eigenvalues, and factor orderings, were supportive of the stability of the eating styles. In response, I identified seven specific overeating styles, and we named them based on the questions that were grouped into a factor.[6]

They are in order of their eigenvalue (strength of item intercorrelation): 1) Sensory Disregard ("flavoring" food with meaning); 2) Emotional Eating (eating to manage feelings); 3) Fast Foodism (eating mostly processed, high-calorie food and less fresh food); 4) Food Fretting (judgmental thoughts and over-concern about food); 5) Task Snacking (eating while doing other activities); 6) Unappetizing Atmosphere (physical and emotional dining environments); 7) and Solo Dining (eating alone versus with others).

The implications of these findings are that when people practice even one of the significant seventy-eight elements, such as eating while working, they are also likely to practice another element in that group, such as eating while reading. This is important when we consider the feasibility of making changes in all seventy-eight elements. In other words, if they are grouped as overeating styles, we believe all behaviors identified with the style can more easily be changed than addressing one element at a time. This thinking supports the philosophy of German sociologist Max Weber, who maintains that when a lifestyle moves from one cultural group to another, it is adopted as a group of elements.[7] This idea was applied to health lifestyles by medical sociologist Thomas Abel, Ph.D., and colleagues.[8]

Demographic considerations. I next considered if the overeating styles we had identified for the total population in our study would hold together similarly for different ages, gender, ethnicity, and education. To assess this, when sample size permitted (for all but ethnicity), I redid the factor analysis within each subgroup. I found the same recurring factor-analytic pattern of the seven eating styles for men and women, by different ages, education levels, and ethnic groups.[6] This means that the questions measuring each perennial theme were similarly interrelated no matter the demographic subgroup. The results supported the validity of the concept of eating styles as well as the universality of these eating styles.

These findings also showed how poorly this large sample were following the ancient-food WPIE guidelines when preparing and eating their meals (66 percent were overweight or obese). Though most were educated and female, they got an overall C grade (on a scale of A to F) on how well they were eating. And as we shall see, when I combined scores for all seven overeating styles, grades worsened with increasing weight. In other words, those with normal weight were about a grade C; those who were overweight were grade D; those who were obese were a D-; and the group of morbidly obese had eating behaviors that scored a grade of F. Clearly there was a linear relationship between weight and the overeating styles: The more participants ate according to the overeating styles, the more overweight; the closer the food choices and eating behaviors were to the perennial WPIE principles, the more normal the weight.

Relationship of eating styles to overeating, overweight, and obesity. At this stage, I did an analysis to see how following the eating styles would predict overeating and weight. **Table 1**, below, shows the bivariate correlations between each eating style and overeating, and the relative strengths of correlations with both overeating and body mass index. I used a linear-regression analysis to find out if these eating styles are independently related to overeating and, if so, how much of the total variance they could predict.

What I discovered was that each of the newly identified overeating styles was independently related to overeating frequency, and together they accounted for over 50 percent of the variance in overeating. That is an impressive result given that these were self-report measures. In the analysis to predict body weight, five of the seven overeating styles were significantly related to overweight and obesity, accounting for a respectable 16 percent of the variance in body mass index (see **Table 2**).

Plots of weight and selected eating behaviors. To obtain a graphic image of the typical relationship between the overeating style questionnaire and weight, I divided the sample of 5,256 into five groups. Then I plotted the mean questionnaire response within each group as the *y*-axis and the weight levels as the *x*-axis. The *y*-axis units correspond to the six-point frequency scale in the questionnaire (*never, rarely, sometimes, usually, almost always, always*).

The three plots below show results from three questions in the questionnaire: "I eat when I am anxious" (**Plot 1**), "I eat processed food" (**Plot 2**), and "I eat fruit" (**Plot 3**). I selected these three questions to show examples of the typical relationship between certain questions and respondents' weight. In plots 1 through 3 you will see substantial differences in eating patterns between every weight grouping (i.e., from underweight to morbidly obese). Notably, the morbidly obese have a poorer relationship with food than the obese, who are worse than the overweight.

Overcoming the overeating styles with Whole Person Integrative Eating. The next question I considered was whether individuals can improve their overeating styles, and if so, would it make a difference in their overeating and weight? In our national sample, the 192 who completed both the pre- and post-overeating styles questionnaire[3] showed improvement in every overeating style. Paired-sample T tests showed a significant reduction in each of the seven eating styles (see **Table 3**). This shows that individuals can indeed make major improvements in their relationship to eating by going from the overeating styles toward Whole Person Integrative Eating guidelines. Other studies done on the WPIE intervention confirm this.[9-12]

But does changing from the overeating styles to Whole Person Integrative Eating make a difference in weight? Yes! The correlation analysis I did measuring changes in the overeating styles and changes in overeating and body mass index show that the more participants changed their eating styles the less they overate and the more weight they lost (see **Table 4**). These results are for a mostly highly motivated subgroup, so while it does not generalize to the general population, it shows that the WPIE model and program guides people to a way of eating that leads to less overeating and more weight loss.

Summary. The research on the overeating styles and Whole Person Integrative Eating provides a strong evidence base for the conceptual framework of the WPIE model and program. In other words, our research supports that the seven overeating styles exist in diverse populations and that each of the styles has an independent relationship to overeating. Also, the validation of the questionnaire provides a useful tool that can be used for teaching and research. Furthermore, initial studies suggest there is short-term evidence that overeating styles can be changed and improved on and that the degree to which one changes is related to the degree to which overeating and weight is lessened.

In other words, our research has revealed that Whole Person Integrative Eating is a sound approach that can improve peoples' relationships to food and eating and in turn their weight. We believe further study is warranted regarding its feasibility and effectiveness in other populations.

Table 1

Cross-Sectional Correlations of Seven Eating Styles with Overeating and Overweight

Eating Style	Stat. Method	Overeating	Body Mass Index
Spiritual Sensory Regard for Food	Pearson Correlation	.318**	-.129**
	Sig. (2-tailed)	.000	.000
	N	5256	1138
Fresh vs Processed Food	Pearson Correlation	.374**	-.284**
	Sig. (2-tailed)	.000	.000
	N	5256	1138
Feelings Prompt Eating	Pearson Correlation	.687**	-.273**
	Sig. (2-tailed)	.000	.000
	N	5256	1138
Food Fretting	Pearson Correlation	.504**	-.145**
	Sig. (2-tailed)	.000	.000
	N	5256	1138
Task Snacking	Pearson Correlation	.275**	-.118**
	Sig. (2-tailed)	.000	.000
	N	5256	1138
Eating Atmosphere	Pearson Correlation	.365**	-.080**
	Sig. (2-tailed)	.000	.007
	N	5256	1138
Eating with Others	Pearson Correlation	.112**	-.110**
	Sig. (2-tailed)	.000	.000
	N	5256	1138
All 7 Eating Styles	Pearson Correlation	.585**	-.252**
	Sig. (2-tailed)	.000	.000
	N	5256	1138

Note: ** indicates significance that is < .001

Table 2
Multiple Regression Analysis of Seven Eating Styles Predicting Reported Overeating and Obesity

Predictor Variables*	Dependent Variables					
	Overeating			Obesity		
	B	t	Prob.	B	t	Prob.
Sensory-Spiritual	.172	18.295	<0.001	-.068	-2.489	0.013
Fresh Food, Fast Food	.224	23.807	<0.001	-.265	-9.708	<0.001
Emotional Eating	.561	59.589	<0.001	-.295	-10.779	<0.001
Food Fretting	.318	33.780	<0.001	.001	.025	0.980
Task-Snacking	.156	16.547	<0.001	-.061	-2.255	0.024
Eating Atmosphere	.119	12.653	<0.001	.057	2.099	0.036
Social Fare	-.028	-3.022	<0.001	-.026	-.949	0.343
Summary Statistics	R^2 = .54			R^2 = .16		
	F (7, 5246) = 862, p <0.001			F (7, 1129) = 31.2, p <0.001		

* Betas are standardized coefficients.

Plot 1
Frequency of Eating when Anxious by Five Weight Levels

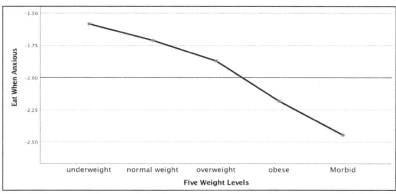

Note: The larger negative score indicates more frequent overeating.

Plot 2
Frequency of Eating Processed Food by Five Weight Levels

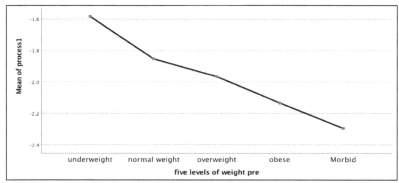

Note: The more negative the score, the higher the frequency of eating processed food.

Plot 3
Frequency of Eating Fruit by Five Weight Levels

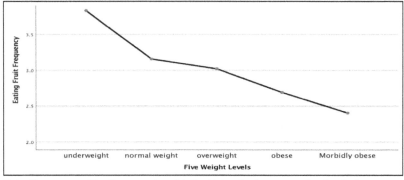

Note: The more positive the score (*y*-axis), the higher the frequency of eating fruit.

Table 3
Mean Differences in Eating Styles After a Six-Week Course

	Pre	Post	St Dev.[a]	t	df	Sig. (2-tailed)
Spiritual Sensory Regard	42.1	54.3	15.8	-12.6	191	p <0.001
Whole or Fast-Food Eating	10.1	16.1	8.3	-13.3	191	p <0.001
Feelings-Prompted Eating	-9.8	-6.5	7.8	-7.2	191	p <0.001
Food Fretting	-19.3	-14.7	8.7	-10.2	191	p <0.001
Emotional Atmosphere	12.8	16.7	5.4	-11.7	191	p <0.001
Eating with Others	4.8	5.6	3.1	-4.6	193	p <0.001
Task Snacking	-6.2	-5.0	3.7	-7.0	193	p <0.001

*For this paired-samples T test, sample size varied from 192 to 194 across the paired comparisons.

[a] The standard deviations are similar for pre and post scores, so only the pre SD is listed.

Table 4
Correlations of Changes in Overeating Styles with Changes in
Overeating and Weight

Pre-Post Changes in Eating Style		Change in Overeating	Change in Weight
Spirit Sensory Change	Pearson Correlation	.338**	.422**
	Sig.	.000	.000
Feelings Prompted Change	Pearson Correlation	.620**	.384**
	Sig.	.000	.000
Emotional Atmosphere Change	Pearson Correlation	.254**	.358**
	Sig.	.000	.000
Eating with Others Change	Pearson Correlation	.192**	.343**
	Sig.	.008	.000
Fresh Fast Food Change	Pearson Correlation	.425**	.326**
	Sig.	.000	.000
Task Snacking Change	Pearson Correlation	.168*	.214*
	Sig.	.020	.016
Neurotic Post-Pre	Pearson Correlation	.457**	.240**
	Sig.	.000	.007
All eating style changes	Pearson Correlation	.522**	.482**
	Sig.	.000	.000

* Less than or equal to .05
** Less than .001

REFERENCES

Introduction: Ancient Food Wisdom Meets Modern Nutritional Science

1. Deborah Kesten, *The Healing Secrets of Food: A Practical Guide for Nourishing Body, Mind, and Soul* (Novato, CA: New World Library, 2001), p. ix.
2. Larry Scherwitz and Deborah Kesten, "Seven Eating Styles Linked to Overeating, Overweight, and Obesity," *Explore: The Journal of Science and Healing* 1, no. 5 (2005): 342–59.
3. Deborah Kesten and Larry Scherwitz, "Whole Person Integrative Eating: A Program for Treating Overeating, Overweight, and Obesity," *Integrative Medicine: A Clinician's Journal* 14, no. 5 (October/November 2015): 42–50.
4. Deborah Kesten and Larry Scherwitz, "What's Your Overeating Style? Self-Assessment Quiz," September 15, 2013, https://www.makeweightlosslast.com/2013/05/06/general-introduction/.

Chapter 1: Discovering Whole Person Integrative Eating

1. D. Riley, "Integrative Nutrition: Food's Multidimensional Power to Heal," *Explore: The Journal of Science and Healing* 1, no. 5 (2005): 340–41.
2. Alison's case study is based on an actual client written about in our research paper, "Whole Person Integrative Eating: A Program for Treating Overeating, Overweight, and Obesity," *Integrative Medicine: A Clinician's Journal*, October 2015. (For the purposes of this book, "Alison" is a composite of an actual client and others I have coached who struggle with weight issues.)
3. Deborah Kesten and Larry Scherwitz, "Whole Person Integrative Eating: A Program for Treating Overeating, Overweight, and Obesity," *Integrative Medicine: A Clinician's Journal* 14, no. 5 (October/November 2015): 42–50.
4. Deborah Kesten, "The Enlightened Diet: Integrating Biological, Spiritual, Social, and Psychological Nutrition," *Spirituality & Health* 5 (2003): 29–39.
5. M. L. Dansinger et al., "Comparison of the Atkins, Ornish, Weight Watchers, and Zone Diets for Weight Loss and Heart Disease Risk Reduction: A Randomized Trial," *Journal of the American Medical Association* 293, no. 1 (2005): 43–53.
6. Daniel DeNoon, "4 Diets Face Off: Which Is the Winner? The Best Diet: The One You Stick With," *WebMd Medical News*, January 4, 2005, www.webmd.com.

7. Larry Scherwitz and Deborah Kesten, "Seven Eating Styles Linked to Overeating, Overweight, and Obesity," *Explore: The Journal of Science and Healing* 1, no. 5 (2005): 342–59.

8. Deborah Kesten and Larry Scherwitz, "What's Your Overeating Style? Self-Assessment Quiz," May 6, 2013, http://www.makeweightlosslast.com/2013/05/06/health-professionals-introduction/.

9. National Center for Health Statistics, Centers for Disease Control and Prevention, "Obesity and Overweight," https://www.cdc.gov/nchs/fastats/obesity-overweight.htm.

10. C.M. Hales, M. Carroll, C. Fryar, and C. Ogden, "Prevalence of Obesity Among Adults and Youth: United States, 2015–2016," NCHS Data Brief, no. 288, U.S. Department of Health and Human Services, Centers for Disease Control and Prevention, https://www.cdc.gov/nchs/data/databriefs/db288.pdf.

11. B. Moss and W. Yeaton, "Young Children's Weight Trajectories and Associated Risk Factors: Results from the Early Childhood Longitudinal Study-Birth Cohort," *American Journal of Health Promotion* 25, no. 3 (2011): 190–8.

12. S. Olshansky et al., "A Potential Decline in Life Expectancy in the United States in the 21st Century," *New England Journal of Medicine* 352, no. 11 (2005): 1138–45.

13. Deborah Kesten, *Feeding the Body, Nourishing the Soul: Essentials of Eating for Physical, Emotional, and Spiritual Well-Being* (Berkeley, CA: Conari Press, 1997; Amherst, MA: White River Press, 2007).

14. Deborah Kesten, *The Healing Secrets of Food: A Practical Guide for Nourishing Body, Mind, and Soul* (Novato, CA: New World Library, 2001).

15. National Center for Health Statistics, Centers for Disease Control and Prevention, "Obesity and Overweight," https://www.cdc.gov/nchs/fastats/obesity-overweight.htm.

16. C.M. Hales et al., "Prevalence of Obesity Among Adults and Youth: United States, 2015–2016," NCHS Data Brief, no. 288, U.S. Department of Health and Human Services, Centers for Disease Control and Prevention, https://www.cdc.gov/nchs/data/databriefs/db288.pdf.

17. Deborah Kesten, "The Enlightened Diet Integrative Eating E-Course." New York: *Spirituality & Health* (December 16, 2002–January 24, 2003).

18. Kelly Brownell, Open Yale Courses, Psychology 123: The Psychology, Biology and Politics of Food, Lecture 2, "Food Then, Food Now: Modern Food Conditions and Their Mismatch with Evolution," accessed March 8, 2012, www.oyc.yale.edu/psychology/psyc-123.

19. Erica Oberg, Ryan Bradley, J. Allen, M. McCrory, "Evaluation of a Naturopathic Nutrition Program for Type 2 Diabetes," *Complementary Therapies and Clinical Practice* 17, no. 3 (2011): 157–61.

20. Ryan Bradley, "Eating Habits and Diabetes: How We Eat May Be More Important Than What We Eat," *Diabetes Action* website, June 2011, www.diabetesaction.org/article-eating-habits?rq=ryan%20bradley%202011.

21. Erin S. Yaseen, M. M. Gehrke, P. Palmer, I. Kavanaugh, B. Walter, T. Reiss, E. Taylor, M. McCroy, "Integrative Eating Style in Relation to Eating Behavior and Adiposity in Healthy Adults," *FASEB Journal* 22, no. 1-supplement (Mar 2008).

22. Deborah Kesten and Larry Scherwitz, "Holistic, Satisfying Meals Key to Optimal Nutrition," *Research News and Opportunities in Science and Theology* 3, no. 3 (2002): 11.

Chapter 2: Meet the Overeating Styles "Family": 7 Root Causes of Overeating

1. Larry Scherwitz and Deborah Kesten, "Seven Eating Styles Linked to Overeating, Over-weight, and Obesity," *Explore: The Journal of Science and Healing* 1, no. 5 (2005): 342–59.

2. The implications of our study are enormous, because not only did we discover new over-eating styles strongly linked with being overweight and obese but we also learned that those who made the most changes in the overeating styles during the study lost the most weight. In other words, the more people improved across all seven overeating styles over the eighteen-week e-course, the more likely they were to lose weight. Perhaps even more inspirational is the realization that motivated research participants made dramatic chang-es in their overeating styles, on their own, by practicing the six-week, eighteen-lesson Whole Person Integrative Eating online e-course.

3. Another contribution of the overeating styles is that they offer a "whole person" per-spective on why so many of us gain weight and struggle with taking and keeping it off. In this way, the overeating styles provide direction for overcoming the various reasons we overeat.

4. Deborah Kesten, *Feeding the Body, Nourishing the Soul: Essentials of Eating for Physical, Emotion-al, and Spiritual Well-Being* (Berkeley, CA: Conari Press, 1997; Amherst, MA: White River Press, 2007).

5. Deborah Kesten, "The Enlightened Diet: Integrating Biological, Spiritual, Social, and Psychological Nutrition," *Spirituality & Health* 5 (2003): 29–39.

6. Deborah Kesten, "The Enlightened Diet Integrative Eating E-Course." New York: *Spiri-tuality & Health* (December 16, 2002–January 24, 2003).

7. Deborah Kesten and Larry Scherwitz, "What's Your Overeating Style? Self-Assess-ment Quiz," May 6, 2013, http://www.makeweightlosslast.com/2013/05/06/health-professionals-introduction/.

8. Deborah Kesten and Larry Scherwitz, "What's Your Overeating Style? Self-Assess-ment Quiz," September 15, 2013, http://www.makeweightlosslast.com/2013/05/06/general-introduction/.

9. Deborah Kesten, *The Healing Secrets of Food: A Practical Guide for Nourishing Body, Mind, and Soul* (Novato, CA: New World Library, 2001).

Chapter 3: What's Your Overeating Style? Self-Assessment Quiz

1. Larry Scherwitz and Deborah Kesten, "Seven Eating Styles Linked to Overeating, Over-weight, and Obesity," *Explore: The Journal of Science and Healing* 1, no. 5 (2005): 342–59.

2. Deborah Kesten and Larry Scherwitz, "Whole Person Integrative Eating: A Program for Treating Overeating, Overweight, and Obesity," *Integrative Medicine: A Clinician's Journal* 14, no. 5 (October/November 2015): 42–50.

3. The seventy-six-item "What's Your Overeating Style?" assessment tool identifies seven eating styles that are linked to overeating, overweight, and obesity. The more elements within each overeating style a person practices, the more likely that person is to overeat and gain weight; conversely, when proactive steps are taken each day to replace the over-eating styles with the Whole Person Integrative Eating dietary lifestyle, odds of fulfilling weight-loss potential increase.

4. The "What's Your Overeating Style? Self-Assessment Quiz" 1) is validated with norms based on a large sample size (N=5,256) 2) and contains seventy-six questions, each of which has been factor analyzed and has shown validity in predicting frequency of overeating.

5. Deborah Kesten, *The Healing Secrets of Food: A Practical Guide for Nourishing Body, Mind, and Soul* (Novato, CA: New World Library, 2001).

6. Deborah Kesten and Larry Scherwitz, "What's Your Overeating Style? Self-Assessment Quiz," May 6, 2013, http://www.makeweightlosslast.com/2013/05/06/health-professionals-introduction/.

7. Deborah Kesten and Larry Scherwitz, "What's Your Overeating Style? Self-Assessment Quiz," September 15, 2013, http://www.makeweightlosslast.com/2013/05/06/general-introduction/.

Chapter 4: Are You Really Ready to Lose Weight?

1. C. DiClemente and J. Prochaska, "Self-change and therapy change of smoking behavior: A comparison of processes of change in cessation and maintenance," *Addictive Behaviors* 7 (1982): 133–42.

2. C. DiClemente, *Addiction and Change: How addictions develop and addicted people recover.* (New York: Guilford Press, 2003).

3. J. Prochaska and C. DiClemente, "Stages and processes of self-change of smoking: Toward an integrative model of change," *Journal of Consulting and Clinical Psychology* 51 (1983): 390–5.

4. J. Prochaska, C. DiClemente, J. Norcross, "In search of how people change: Applications to addictive behaviors," *American Psychologist* 47 (1992): 1102–14.

5. B. Marcus, S. Banspach, R. Lefebvre, J. Rossi, R. Carleton, and D. Abrams, "Using the stages of change model to increase the adoption of physical activity among community participants," *American Journal of Health Promotion* 6 (1992): 424–29.

6. C. Nigg, P. Burbank, C. Padula, R. Dufresne, J. Rossi, W. Velicer, R. Laforge, and J. Prochaska, "Stages of change across ten health risk behaviors for older adults," *The Gerontologist* 39 (1999): 473–82.

7. R. Westermeyer, "A User-Friendly Model of Change," Habit Smart, September 5, 2005, www.habitsmart.com/motivate.htm.

Chapter 5: What's a Dietary Lifestyle, Anyway? (Hint: Overeating Styles Rx)

1. Roxanne Swentzell and Patricia M. Perea, eds., *The Pueblo Food Experience Cookbook: Whole Food of Our Ancestors* (New Mexico: Museum of New Mexico Press, 2016).

2. Inez Russell Gomez, "Artist Reclaims Native Culture with Ancestral Foods," *The New Mexican*, accessed August 30, 2018, http://www.santafenewmexican.com/news/community/artist-reclaims-native-culture-with-ancestral-foods/article_21a8e264-1c29-5e25-b0f4-e384a643a2af.html.

3. Deon Ben, "Food as Medicine: The Healing Power of Native foods," Grand Canyon Trust, December 9, 2016, https://www.grandcanyontrust.org/blog/food-medicine-healing-power-native-foods.

4. D. McLaughlin, "The Pueblo Food Experience," Vimeo.com, December 29, 2013.

5. Ayto J., *Dictionary of Word Origins* (New York: Little, Brown and Company, 1990).

6. English Oxford Living Dictionary, accessed September 1, 2018, https://en.oxforddictionaries.com/definition/diet.

7. Dean Ornish, Larry Scherwitz, J. Billings, L. Gould, T. Merritt, and S. Sparler, "The Impact of Major Lifestyle Changes on Coronary Stenosis, CHD Risk Factors, and Psychological Status: Results from the San Francisco Lifestyle Heart Trial." *Progression and Regression of Atherosclerosis*. Proceedings of a Symposium dedicated to David H. Blankenhorn. (Koenig W, Hombach V, Bond M, Kramsch D, editors) Blackwell-MZV, Vienna, (1995).

8. Dean Ornish, Larry Scherwitz, J. Billings, et al., "Can Intensive Lifestyle Changes Reverse Coronary Heart Disease Without Lipid-Lowering Drugs? Five-Year Follow-up of the Lifestyle Heart Trial," *Journal of the American Medical Association* 280, no. 23, (1998): 201–8.

9. Dean Ornish, S. Brown, Larry Scherwitz, et al., "Can Lifestyle Changes Reverse Coronary Heart Disease?" *The Lancet* 336, no. 8708 (1990): 129–33.

10. Jeffrey Bland, accessed March 2, 2019, https://jeffreybland.com.

11. Larry Scherwitz and Deborah Kesten, "Seven Eating Styles Linked to Overeating, Overweight, and Obesity," *Explore: The Journal of Science and Healing* 1, no. 5 (2005): 342–59.

12. Deborah Kesten and Larry Scherwitz, "What's Your Overeating Style? Self-Assessment Quiz," May 6, 2013, http://www.makeweightlosslast.com/2013/05/06/health-professionals-introduction/.

13. Deborah Kesten and Larry Scherwitz, "What's Your Overeating Style? Self-Assessment Quiz," September 15, 2013, http://www.makeweightlosslast.com/2013/05/06/general-introduction/.

14. Deborah Kesten and Larry Scherwitz, "Whole Person Integrative Eating: A Program for Treating Overeating, Overweight, and Obesity," *Integrative Medicine: A Clinician's Journal* 14, no. 5 (October/November 2015): 42–50.

Chapter 6: Emotional Eating Rx: Positive Feelings

1. A. Dingemans, U. Danner, M. Parks, "Emotion Regulation in Binge Eating Disorder: A Review," *Nutrients* 9, no. 11 (2017): 1274.

2. Larry Scherwitz and Deborah Kesten, "Seven Eating Styles Linked to Overeating, Overweight, and Obesity," *Explore: The Journal of Science and Healing* 1, no. 5 (2005): 342–59.

3. A correlational analysis of emotionally based overeating reveals that all negative emotions are equally and strongly correlated with overeating. Note the correlations: "I eat because I feel" anxious ($r=.55$), frustrated ($r=.55$), depressed ($r=.55$), sad ($r=.53$), angry ($r=.52$), craving ($r=.52$); the positive emotion of happy ($r=.29$) was least correlated with overeating.

4. Our research on the overeating styles revealed that those who reported overeating more frequently were significantly more likely to eat when they were sad, depressed, angry, frustrated, anxious, or experiencing food cravings. *Check in with hunger level:* the more participants check their hunger level before eating, the less likely they are to overeat; ($r=.41$); while those who "check in" and only eat when they are hungry are also less likely to overeat ($r=.50$). Those who check their hunger level are also less likely to be obese ($r=-.20$). *Eat only when hungry:* if participants eat only when they are hungry, they are thinner, less likely to be obese ($r=-.22$), and less likely to be overweight ($r=-.22$); conversely, if participants eat regardless of whether they're hungry, they will weigh more ($r=-.22$).

5. Deborah Kesten, "The enlightened diet integrative eating e-course," New York: *Spirituality & Health* (December 16, 2002–January 24, 2003).

6. Deborah Kesten, "The enlightened diet: integrating biological, spiritual, social, and psychological nutrition," *Spirituality & Health* (2003): 29–39.

7. The 102 highly motivated individuals who completed the same overeating style questionnaire both before and after completing the Whole Person Integrative Eating online course had a significant reduction in all five of the individual negative feelings; they also had a significant reduction in their overeating frequency. In a further analysis, we found that those who reduced their negative feelings the most were likely to switch their food choices from eating processed, fried food, and sweets to eating more legumes and vegetables. The combination of reducing negative feelings and improved food choices were correlated with how much weight these individuals lost, so we think that feelings and food choices are key factors in controlling weight.

8. Deborah Kesten and Larry Scherwitz, "Holistic, satisfying meals key to optimal nutrition," *Research News and Opportunities in Science and Theology* 3, no. 3 (2002): 11.

9. Deborah Kesten and Larry Scherwitz, "What's Your Overeating Style? Self-Assessment Quiz," May 6, 2013, http://www.makeweightlosslast.com/2013/05/06/health-professionals-introduction/.

10. Deborah Kesten and Larry Scherwitz, "Whole Person Integrative Eating: A Program for Treating Overeating, Overweight, and Obesity," *Integrative Medicine: A Clinician's Journal* 14, no. 5 (October/November 2015): 42–50.

11. Erica Oberg, Ryan Bradley, J. Allen, and M. McCrory, "Evaluation of a naturopathic nutrition program for type 2 diabetes," *Complementary Therapies in Clinical Practice* 17, no. 3 (2011): 157–61.

12. Ryan Bradley, "Eating habits and diabetes: how we eat may be more important than what we eat," *Diabetes Action* website, June 2011, www.diabetesaction.org/article-eating-habits?rq=ryan%20bradley%202011.

13. Erica Oberg, e-mail to co-author Larry Scherwitz, September 7, 2018.

14. Overeaters Anonymous, accessed December 8, 2006, www.oa.org/lifeline_monthly.html.

15. Judith J. Wurtman, *Managing Your Mind and Mood through Food* (New York: Rawson Associates, 1986).

16. V. Cardi, J. Leppanen, and J.Treasure, "The effects of negative and positive mood induction on eating behaviour: A meta-analysis of laboratory studies in the healthy population and eating and weight disorders," *Neurosci Biobehav Rev.* 57 (Oct 2015): 299–309.

17. Human Microbiome Project, *The NIH Common Fund.* https://commonfund.nih.gov/hmp, retrieved September 10, 2018.

18. J. Cryan, S. O'Mahony, "The microbiome-gut-brain axis: from bowel to behavior," *Neurogastroenterology Motility* 23 (2011): 187–92.

19. L. Goehler, M. Lyte, R. Gaykema, "Infection-induced viscerosensory signals from the gut enhance anxiety: implications for psychoneuroimmunology," *Brain Behavior and Immunology* 21 (2007): 721–6.

20. J. Cryan, T. Dinan, "Mind-altering microorganisms: the impact of the gut microbiota on brain and behavior," *Nature Reviews Neuroscience*, 13 (October 2012): 701–12.

21. M. Pinto-Sanchez, "Probiotic Bifidobacterium longum Reduces Depression Scores and Alters Brain Activity: A Pilot Study in Patients with Irritable Bowel Syndrome,"*Gastroenterology* 153, no. 2 (August 2017): 448–459.

22. Anxiety and Depression Association of America, "Facts and Statistics," accessed September 13, 2018, https://adaa.org/about-adaa/press-room/facts-statistics.

23. S. Manfredo Vieira, M. Hiltensperger, V. Kumar, D. Zegarra-Ruiz, et al., "Translocation of a gut pathobiont drives autoimmunity in mice and humans," *Science* 359, no. 6380 (2018): 1156.

24. B. Watzl, "Anti-inflammatory effects of plant-based foods and of their constituents," *Int J Vitam Nutr Res* 78, no. 6 (2008): 293–8.

25. Deborah Kesten, *"Whole Person Integrative Eating (WPIE) Guided Meal Meditation: Creating Conscious Connection to Overcome Your Overeating Styles,"* January 28, 2013, https://www.makeweightlosslast.com/2013/01/28/free-audio-wpie-guided-meal-meditation/.

Chapter 7: Food Fretting Rx: Appreciate Food

1. Jack Kornfield, "Gratitude and Wonder," accessed September 18, 2018, https://jackkornfield.com/gratitude/.

2. Obsessing about food is the "umbrella" that links all ten Food Fretting thoughts, feelings, and behaviors: counting calories, feeling anxiety about the "best" way to eat, feeling gluttonous, bad, and guilty when overeating, obsessing about food, dieting, judging others' food choices and eating behaviors, and feeling righteous when eating what one "should."

3. Deborah Kesten, "The enlightened diet integrative eating e-course." New York: *Spirituality & Health* (December 16, 2002–January 24, 2003).

4. Deborah Kesten and Larry Scherwitz, "What's Your Overeating Style? Self-Assessment Quiz," September 15, 2013, http://www.makeweightlosslast.com/2013/05/06/general-introduction.

5. Could the Whole Person Integrative Eating e-course help reduce Food Fretting and in turn lower odds of overeating and weight gain? The 192 individuals who took the course *and* completed the pre- and post-overeating styles questionnaire made substantial improvements of from 1 to 2.7 points on the 5-point scale in the Food Fretting eating style items. The pre-post comparisons using a paired samples T test were significant to beyond <0.001 for all ten items!

6. The Food Fretting factors most related to overeating were craving food (r = .51, p >0.001), feeling bad (r = .41), feeling guilty (r = .53), or gluttonous (r = .44) after overeating, and obsessing about food (r = .54).

7. Larry Scherwitz and Deborah Kesten, "Seven Eating Styles Linked to Overeating, Overweight, and Obesity," *Explore: The Journal of Science and Healing* 1, no. 5 (2005): 342–59.

8. "Three Out Of Four American Women Have Disordered Eating, Survey Suggests," *Science News*, accessed September 18, 2011, http://www.sciencedaily.com/releases/2008/04/080422202514.htm.

9. National Association of Eating Disorders, accessed September 17, 2018, www.nationaleatingdisorders.org/index.php.

10. U.S. Department of Health and Human Services, "Rate of Eating Disorders in Kids Keeps Rising," accessed July 18, 2011, http://www.healthfinder.gov/news/newsstory.aspx?docID=646574.

11. Sarah Kaplan, "Psychiatry doesn't recognize 'orthorexia'—an obsession with healthy eating. But the Internet does," *The Washington Post*, November 5, 2015, https://www.washingtonpost.com/news/morning-mix/wp/2015/11/05/psychiatry-doesnt-recognize-orthorexia-an-obsession-with-healthy-eating-but-the-internet-does/?utm_term=.ddaa30819265.

12. NEDA, "Orthorexia," NationalEatingDisorders.org, accessed October 20, 2018, https://www.nationaleatingdisorders.org/learn/by-eating-disorder/other/orthorexia.

13. Deborah Kesten and Larry Scherwitz, "Whole Person Integrative Eating: A Program for Treating Overeating, Overweight, and Obesity," *Integrative Medicine: A Clinician's Journal* 14, no. 5 (October/November 2015): 42–50.

14. Deborah Kesten, *The Healing Secrets of Food: A Practical Guide for Nourishing Body, Mind, and Soul* (Novato, CA: New World Library, 2001).

15. Michael Mayer, Ph.D. (clinical psychologist), phone interview with Deborah Kesten, San Francisco, California.

16. Ayo Ngozi, "Gladdening the Heart: Historical Perspectives and Therapeutics," *Journal of the American Herbalists Guild* 11, no. 1 (2016): 47–55. http://www.ayongozi.com/wp-content/uploads/2016/11/Gladdening-1.pdf.

17. Larry Scherwitz, "Type A behavior, self-involvement, and coronary atherosclerosis," *Psychosomatic Medicine* 45, no.1 (1983): 47–57.

18. Doc Lew Childre and Howard Martin, *The HeartMath Solution* (San Francisco: HarperSanFrancisco, 2000).

19. HeartMath Institute: Science of the Heart, "Exploring the Role of the Heart in Human Performance: An Overview of Research Conducted by the HeartMath Institute," accessed September 18, 2018, https://www.heartmath.org/research/science-of-the-heart/energetic-communication/.

20. Deborah Kesten, "Saying Grace," *Yoga Journal* (September/October 2001): 49–53.

Chapter 8: Fast Foodism Rx: Get Fresh

1. Michael Pollan, *The Omnivore's Dilemma: A Natural History of Four Meals* (London: Bloomsbury Publishing Plc, 2006).

2. Mark Hyman, "Systems Biology: The Gut-Brain-Fat Cell Connection and Obesity," *Alternative Therapies* 12, no. 1 (2006): 10.

3. Larry Scherwitz and Deborah Kesten, "Seven Eating Styles Linked to Overeating, Overweight, and Obesity," *Explore: The Journal of Science and Healing* 1, no. 5 (2005): 342–59.

4. Deborah Kesten and Larry Scherwitz, "What's Your Overeating Style? Self-Assessment Quiz," September 15, 2013, http://www.makeweightlosslast.com/2013/05/06/general-introduction/.

5. Judith C. Rodriguez, "Fast Foods Health," *Gale Encyclopedia of Nutrition and Well Being* (New York: Gale Group, 2004), www.healthline.com/galecontent/fast-foods.

6. Yourdictionary.com, "junk food," September 18, 2018, www.yourdictionary.com/junk-food.

7. Bridget Murray, "Fast-Food Culture Serves Up Super-Size Americans," *Monitor on Psychology* 32, no. 11 (2001): www.apa.org/monitor/dec01/fastfood.html.

8. All seven overeating styles are statistically correlated with overeating frequency (p <0.001), and five of the seven are correlated with weight (p <0.02). The Fast Foodism overeating style ranked third for its link to overeating. The Emotional Eating and Food Fretting overeating styles ranked numbers 1 and 2 respectively, for overeating. The strongest overeating-style predictors for obesity were Emotional Eating, Fast Foodism, and Sensory Disregard (all significant to p <0.02).

9. Georgia Jones, "Fast Foods! A 4-H Lifelong Learning Resource," *Journal of Nutrition Education and Behavior* 38, no. 4 (2006): supplement S37; B. Liebman, "The Pressure to Eat," *Nutrition Action*, July/August 1998: www.cspinet.org/nah/7_98eat.htm; "Fast Food," Wikipedia, accessed December 5, 2006: www.en.wikipedia.org/wiki/Fast_food; D. Mozaffarian, M. Katan, A. Ascherio, M. Stampfer, and W. C. Willett, "Trans Fatty Acids and Cardiovascular Disease," *New England Journal of Medicine* 354, no. 1 (2006): 1601–13; F. Hu, R. van Dam, and S. Liu, "Diet and Risk of Type II Diabetes: The Role of Types of Fat and Carbohydrate," *Diabetologia* 44, no. 7 (2001): 805–17; R. van Dam, M. Stamp-

fer, W. Willett, F. Hu, and E. Rimm, "Dietary Fat and Meat Intake in Relation to Risk of Type 2 Diabetes in Men," *Diabetes Care* 25, no. 3 (2002): 417–24; A. Gosline, "Why Fast Foods Are Bad, Even in Moderation," *New Scientist*, June 12, 2006, https://www .newscientist.com/article/dn9318-why-fast-foods-are-bad-even-in-moderation/.

10. Deborah Kesten, *The Healing Secrets of Food: A Practical Guide for Nourishing Body, Mind, and Soul* (Novato, CA: New World Library, 2001).

11. G. Ma, Y. Li, Y. Wu, F. Zhai, Z. Cui, X. Hu, et al., "The Prevalence of Body Overweight and Obesity and Its Changes among Chinese People during 1992 to 2002," *Chinese Journal of Preventive Medicine* 39 (2005): 311–15 (in Chinese, with English abstract); Y. Wu, G. Ma, Y. Hu, Y. Li, X. Li, Z. Cui, et al., "The Current Prevalence Status of Body Overweight and Obesity in China: Data from the China Nutrition and Health Survey," *Chinese Journal of Preventive Medicine* 39 (2005): 316–20 (in Chinese, with English abstract).

12. France24.com, "French childhood obesity trends downward as global rates rise," December 2, 2017, https://www.france24.com/en/20170212-french-childhood-obesity-trends -downward-global-rates-rise-france.

13. "McDonald's USA Ingredients Listing for Popular Menu Items," accessed September 18, 2018, http://s3.amazonaws.com/us-east-prod-dep-share-s3/dna/pushlive /ingredientslist.pdf.

14. Michael Lueck and Kim Severson, "New York Bans Most Trans Fats in Restaurants," *New York Times*, December 6, 2006, https://www.nytimes.com/2006/12/06/nyregion /06fat.html.

15. Nicholas Bakalar, "Trans Fat Bans Tied to Fewer Heart Attacks and Strokes," *New York Times*, April 12, 2017, https://www.nytimes.com/2017/04/12/well/eat/trans-fat-bans -tied-to-fewer-heart-attacks-and-strokes.html.

16. Brian Hoffmann, "The Influence of Sugar and Artificial Sweeteners on Vascular Health during the Onset and Progression of Diabetes," *Experimental Biology*, accessed September 23, 2018, https://plan.core-apps.com/eb2018/abstract/382e0c7eb95d6e76976fbc663612d58a.

17. "Sugar: Sweet by Nature," advertisement, *News Tribune*, Tacoma, WA, (December 7, 2006).

18. McDonalds.com, accessed September 20, 2018, https://www.mcdonalds.com/gb /en-gb/help/faq/19077-how-many-carbs-are-in-a-happy-meal-with-hamburger-and -coca-cola.html.

19. Mark Hyman, "5 Reasons Why High Fructose Corn Syrup Will Kill You," DrHyman.com, accessed September 21, 2018, https://drhyman.com/blog/2011/05 /13/5-reasons-high-fructose-corn-syrup-will-kill-you.

20. L. Christopher, J. Uribarri, and K. Tucker, "Intake of high fructose corn syrup sweetened soft drinks, fruit drinks and apple juice is associated with prevalent coronary heart disease, in U.S. adults, ages 45–59 y," *BMC Nutrition*, 14:107, June 27, 2017.

21. Anna Gosline, "Why Fast Foods Are Bad, Even in Moderation," *New Scientist*, June 12, 2006, https://www.newscientist.com/article/dn9318-why-fast-foods-are-bad-even-in -moderation/.

22. F. Hu, R. van Dam, and S. Liu, "Diet and Risk of Type II Diabetes: The Role of Types of Fat and Carbohydrate," *Diabetologia* 44, no. 7 (2001): 805–17.

23. A. Krishnan, P. Stathis, S. F. Permuth, et al., "Bisphenol-A: An Estrogenic Substance Is Released from Polycarbonate Flasks During Autoclaving," *Endocrinology* 132, no. 6 (1993): 2279–86.

24. Breast Cancer Fund, "Chemicals in Plastics," accessed February 6, 2012, http://www .breastcancerfund.org/clear-science/chemicals-linked-to-breast-cancer/plastics/.

25. I. Lang, T. Galloway, A. Scarlett, et al., "Association of Urinary Bisphenol A Concentration with Medical Disorders and Laboratory Abnormalities in Adults," *The Journal of the American Medical Association* 300, no. 11 (2008): 1303–10.

26. R. Stahlhut, E. van Wijngaarden, T. Dye, et al., "Concentrations of Urinary Phthalate Metabolites Are Associated with Increased Waist Circumference and Insulin Resistance in Adult U.S. Males," *Environmental Health Perspectives* 115, no. 6 (2007): 876–82.

27. D. LeeI, K. Lee, H. Jin, et al., "Association between Serum Concentrations of Persistent Organic Pollutants and Insulin Resistance among Nondiabetic Adults: Results from the National Health and Nutrition Examination Survey 1999–2002," *Diabetes Care* 30, no. 3 (2007): 622–8.

28. O. Vasiliu, L. Cameron, J. Gardiner, et al., "Polybrominated Biphenyls, Polychlorinated Biphenyls, Body Weight, and Incidence of Adult-Onset Diabetes Mellitus," *Epidemiology* 17, no. 4 (2006): 352–9.

29. H. Masuno, T. Kidani, K. Sekiya, et al., "Bisphenol A in Combination with Insulin Can Accelerate the Conversion of 3T3-L1 Fibroblasts to Adipocytes," *Journal of Lipid Research* 43, no. 5 (2002): 676–84.

30. F. Grün, H. Watanabe, Z. Zamanian, et al., "Endocrine-Disrupting Organotin Compounds Are Potent Inducers of Adipogenesis in Vertebrates," *Molecular Endocrinology* 20, no. 9 (2006): 2141–55.

31. CBC News, Health, "Years of Exposure to BPA Linked to Health Risks in Humans," September 16, 2008, http://www.cbc.ca/news/health/story/2008/09/15/bpa-jama .html.

32. C. Dyer, "Heavy Metals as Endocrine Disrupting Chemicals," in *Endocrine Disrupting Chemicals: From Basic Research to Clinical Practice*, ed. A.C. Gore (Totowa, NJ: Humana Press, 2007), 111–33.

33. Leah Zerbe, "BPA to Be Banned by Congress," May 17, 2010, www.rodale.com/bpa -and-health-risks.

34. Dean Ornish, *Eat More, Weigh Less: Dr. Dean Ornish's Life Choice Program for Losing Weight Safely while Eating Abundantly* (New York: HarperCollins, 1993).

35. P. Turnbaugh, "Gut Microbiota and Obesity," *Cellular and Molecular Life Sciences* 73, no. 1 (October 2015): 213–23.

36. P. Turnbaugh, F. Bäckhed, L. Fulton, and J. Gordon, "Diet-induced obesity is linked to marked but reversible alterations in the mouse distal gut microbiome," *Cell Host Microbe* 3, no. 4 (2008): 213–223.

37. P. Maruvada, V. Leone, L. Kaplan, and E. Chang, "The Human Microbiome and Obesity: Moving beyond Associations," *Cell Host and Microbe* 22, no. 5 (2017): 589–99.

38. Jillian Levy, "The Human Microbiome: How It Works + a Diet for Gut Health: Foods to Eat," draxe.com, January 7, 2016.

39. K. Neufeld, N. Kang, J. Bienenstock, J. Foster, "Reduced anxiety-like behavior and central neurochemical change in germ-free mice," *Neurogastroenterol Motil* 23 (2010): 255–64.

Chapter 9: Sensory Disregard Rx: Nourish Your Senses

1. Jean Anthelme Brillat-Savarin, "On the Pleasures of the Table," *The Physiology of Taste* (New York: Alfred A. Knopf, 1949), 183.

2. Deborah Kesten, *Feeding the Body, Nourishing the Soul: Essentials of Eating for Physical, Emotional, and Spiritual Well-Being* (Berkeley, CA: Conari Press, 1997; Amherst, MA: White River Press, 2007).

3. Larry Scherwitz and Deborah Kesten, "Seven Eating Styles Linked to Overeating, Overweight, and Obesity," *Explore: The Journal of Science and Healing* 1, no. 5 (2005): 342–59.

4. Deborah Kesten and Larry Scherwitz, "What's Your Overeating Style? Self-Assessment Quiz," September 15, 2013, http://www.makeweightlosslast.com/2013/05/06/general-introduction/.

5. Deborah Kesten, "The enlightened diet integrative eating e-course." New York: *Spirituality & Health* (December 16, 2002–January 24, 2003).

6. The 126 individuals who completed both the pre- and post-overeating styles questionnaire and took the six-week, eighteen-lesson e-course significantly and substantially improved on each of the eighteen nourish-your-senses items (all p's <0.001). This group was clearly the most motivated; our results show what motivated people can accomplish re curtailing overeating and weight loss.

7. The statistical method we used, called factor analysis, paired the sensory-spiritual "ingredients" into one overeating style. Our correlational analysis revealed that the more each of these eighteen items are practiced, the less likely participants are to overeat. All eighteen of these correlations with overeating were significant to less than 0.001; the three most strongly correlated are planning meals with care (r=.28) and appreciation (r=.27) and eating with the senses by savoring the scents of food (r=.29). All but one of the remaining food-related items were correlated above r=2, consistently showing that the more participants practiced a spiritual sensual approach to food preparation and eating, the less they ate. While we cannot conclusively state a causal relationship, the results suggest that incorporating spiritual and sensual elements into the dining experience may be an effective way to curtail overeating.

8. Namgyal Qusar, First International Conference on Tibetan Medicine, Washington, DC, November 7–9, 1998.

9. Deborah Kesten, *Feeding the Body, Nourishing the Soul: Essentials of Eating for Physical, Emotional, and Spiritual Well-Being* (Berkeley, CA: Conari Press, 1997; Amherst, MA: White River Press, 2007).

10. R. de Wijk, I. Polet, W. Boek, S. Coenraad, and H. Johannes, "Food aroma affects bite size," *Flavour* 1 (March 20, 2012): 3.

11. R. Estruch, E. Ros, J. Salas-Salvadó, et al., "Primary prevention of cardiovascular disease with a Mediterranean diet," *N Engl J Med* (2013): 368, 1279–1290.

12. M. de Lorgeril, "Reduction in the incidence of type 2 diabetes with the Mediterranean diet," *Diabetes Care* 34, no. 1 (2011): 14–9.

13. José Manuel Fernández-Real, Mónica Bulló, et al., "A Mediterranean Diet Enriched with Olive Oil Is Associated with Higher Serum Total Osteocalcin Levels in Elderly Men at High Cardiovascular Risk," *The Journal of Clinical Endocrinology & Metabolism* 97, no. 10 (2012): 3792–3798.

14. J. Perona, J. Cañizares, E. Montero, et al., "Virgin olive oil reduces blood pressure in hypertensive elderly subjects," *Clinical Nutrition* 23 no. 5 (2004): 1113–21.

15. P. Cohen, "Olive oil may reduce breast cancer risk," *New Scientist* 185, no. 2482 (2005): 7.

16. C. Razquin, J. Martinez, M. Martinez-Gonzalez, et al., "A 3-year follow-up of a Mediterranean diet rich in virgin olive oil is associated with high plasma antioxidant capacity and reduced body weight gain," *Eur J Clin Nutr.* 63, no. 12 (2009): 1387–93.

17. P. Schieberle, V. Somoza, M. Rubach, L. Scholl, and M. Balzer, Identifying substances that regulate satiety in oils and fats and improving low-fat foodstuffs by adding lipid compounds with a high satiety effect; Key findings of the DFG/AiF cluster project "Perception of fat content and regulating satiety: an approach to developing low-fat foodstuffs," 2009–2012.

18. Anahad O'Connor, "Is the Secret to Olive Oil in Its Scent?" *The New York Times*, Health-Science, March 29, 2013, http://well.blogs.nytimes.com/2013/03/29/is-the-secret-to-olive-oil-in-its-scent/.

19. P. Schieberle, "Olive Oil Makes You Feel Full," *Research News*, Technical University of Munich, (March 14, 2013).

20. R. Nerem, J. Murina, J. Levesque, and J. Cornhill, "Social Environment as a Factor in Diet-Induced Atherosclerosis," *Science New Series* 208, no. 4451 (1980): 1475–76.

21. Deepak Chopra, *Body, Mind and Soul*, PBS, KQED-TV, San Francisco, March 7, 1995.

22. Michael Mayer (Ph.D., psychologist, Orinda, CA), conversation with Deborah Kesten, December 5,1996.

Chapter 10: Task Snacking Rx: Mindfulness Eating

1. Souray Adhikari, "Top 33 Mindful and Peaceful Jon Kabat-Zinn Quotes," May 17, 2016, https://indihope.com/2016/05/17/33-mindfulness-quotes-from-jon-kabat-zinn/.

2. Nanci Hellmich and Jo dee Black, "Desktop dining: recipe for disaster," *Great Falls Tribune*, March 1, 2004, www.greatfallstribune.com/news/stories/20040301/localnews/49568.html.

3. Healthwatch, "Car Cuisine: Food Industry Caters to Drivers Eating Behind the Wheel," *CBS News*, November 9, 2005, www.cbsnews.com/stories/2005/11/09/health/main1029857.shtml.

4. The Task Snacking correlations are all statistically significant (p <.001), but are correlated with overeating to a modest degree. Four of the eight items have correlations in the r = −0.20 to −0.23 range, and four have correlations in the −.12 and −.18 range.

5. When we asked whether task snackers overate, we discovered that frequent overeating was linked with all of the seven Task Snacking items. All eight overeating behaviors were statistically significant, though only to a modest degree (p <.001), but they are correlated with overeating to a modest degree. Four of the eight items have correlations in the r = −0.20 to −0.23 range, and four have correlations in the −.12 and −.18 range.

6. We asked whether individuals can reduce Task Snacking behaviors by taking our six-week, eighteen-lesson, Whole Person Integrative Eating e-course. A paired-samples T test showed all seven Task Snacking behaviors to be slightly to moderately reduced after six weeks; all exceed the p <.001 threshold.

7. Larry Scherwitz, Deborah Kesten, O. Brusis, et al., "Are Comprehensive Lifestyle Changes Possible in German Heart Patients?" Pilot study findings. *Progression and Regression of Atherosclerosis*, W. Koenig, V. Hombach, M. Bond, D. Kramsch, editors (Vienna: Blackwell-MZV, 1995).

8. Dean Ornish, Larry Scherwitz, Rochelle Doody, Deborah Kesten, et al., "Effects of Stress Management Training and Dietary Changes in Treating Ischemic Heart Disease," *Journal of the American Medical Association* 249, no. 1 (1983): 54–9.

9. Mindful Staff, "Jon Kabat-Zinn: Defining Mindfulness," Mindful.org, January 11, 2017, https://www.mindful.org/jon-kabat-zinn-defining-mindfulness/.

10. D. Morse and M. Furst, "Meditation: An In-depth Study," *Journal of the American Society of Psychosomatic Dentistry and Medicine* 29, no. 5 (1982): 1–96.

11. Jean Kristeller, "An Exploratory Study of a Meditation-Based Intervention for Binge Eating Disorder," *Journal of Health Psychology* 4, no. 3 (1999): 357–63.

12. Jean Kristeller, "Know Your Hunger," *Spirituality & Health* 8, no. 2 (2005).

13. Dean Ornish, S. Brown, Larry Scherwitz, et al., "Can Lifestyle Changes Reverse Coronary Heart Disease? The Lifestyle Heart Trial," *The Lancet* 336, no. 8708 (1990): 129–33.

14. J. Daubenmier, G. Weidner, M. Sumner, N. Mendell, et al., "The Contribution of Changes in Diet, Exercise, and Stress Management to Changes in Coronary Risk in Women and Men in the Multisite Cardiac Lifestyle Intervention Program," *Annals of Behavioral Medicine* 33 (January 2007) 57–68.

15. Gerdi Weidner (Ph.D., vice president and director of research, Preventive Medicine Research Institute, Sausalito, CA), conversation with Deborah Kesten, October 20, 2006.

16. G. Jacobs, "The Physiology of Mind-Body Interactions: The Stress Response and the Relaxation Response," *Journal of Alternative and Complementary Medicine* 8, no. 2 (2004): supplement 1: https://doi.org/10.1089/1075553.

17. R. Davidson, "Alterations in Brain and Immune Function Produced by Mindfulness Meditation," *Psychosomatic Medicine* 66, no. 1 (2004): 147–52.

18. Herbert Benson, *The Relaxation Response* (New York: William Morrow, 1975).

19. Deborah Kesten, *Feeding the Body, Nourishing the Soul: Essentials of Eating for Physical, Emotional, and Spiritual Well-Being* (Berkeley, CA: Conari Press, 1997; Amherst, MA: White River Press, 2007).

20. Urasenke Foundation, *The Urasenke Tradition of Chado* (Kyoto, Japan: Urasenke Foundation, 1995).

21. Deborah Kesten, *Feeding the Body, Nourishing the Soul: Essentials of Eating for Physical, Emotional, and Spiritual Well-Being* (Berkeley, CA: Conari Press, 1997; Amherst, MA: White River Press, 2007), 204–207.

Chapter 11: Unappetizing Atmosphere Rx: Amiable Ambiance

1. Deborah Kesten and Larry Scherwitz, "What's Your Overeating Style? Self-Assessment Quiz," September 15, 2013, http://www.makeweightlosslast.com/2013/05/06/general-introduction/.

2. A paired-samples T Test showed a significant and substantial improvement in each of the seven elements, with all f ratios exceeding 5.7, p <.001.

3. Feelings of relaxation after eating was the strongest negative correlate (r = .30) of overeating, followed closely by feeling calm after eating (r = .28). Those who lost the most weight were more likely to have more fun while preparing food (r = .23) and be more calm (r = .31) and relaxed (r = .34) after eating.

4. These correlations are relatively strong ranging from r = .40 to .80. When food is prepared in a pleasing, amiable atmosphere individuals tend to overeat less often (r = .22, p <.001).

5. Those who reported preparing food in a more serene and less tense atmosphere also were likely to overeat less often (r = .27 and r = .19 respectively).

6. Those who lost the most weight were more likely to have more fun while preparing food (r = .23) and be more calm (r = .31) and relaxed (r = .34) after eating.

7. E. Widdowson, "Mental Contentment and Physical Growth," *The Lancet* 1, no. 24 (June 16, 1951): 1316–18.

8. Reginald Horsman, *Frontier Doctor William Beaumont, America's First Great Medical Scientist* (Columbia, MO: University of Missouri Press, 1996).

9. C. Pert, S. Snyder, "Opiate receptor: demonstration in nervous tissue," *Science* 179, no. 4077 (March 1973): 1011–4.

10. Candace B. Pert, *Molecules of Emotion: Why You Feel the Way You Feel* (New York: Scribner, 1997), 297–98.

11. N. Garg, B. Wansink, and J. Jeffrey, "The Influence of Incidental Affect on Consumers' Food Intake," *Journal of Marketing* 71, no. 1 (2007), 194.

12. W. Jonas and R. Chez, "Toward optimal healing environments in health care," *J Altern Complement Med*, 2004; 10 Suppl 1:S1-6, https://www.ncbi.nlm.nih.gov/pubmed/15630817.

13. M. Schweitzer, L. Gilpin, S. Frampton, "Healing Spaces: Elements of Environmental Design That Make an Impact on Health," *The Journal of Alternative and Complementary Medicine,* 10 (2004), supplement 1: S71–S83.

14. Christine Aaron, "Anti-Aging Breakthroughs," conversation with author Mireille Guiliano and Oprah Winfrey, *The Oprah Winfrey Show,* May 17, 2005.

15. Larry Scherwitz and Deborah Kesten, "Seven Eating Styles Linked to Overeating, Overweight, and Obesity," *Explore: The Journal of Science and Healing* 1, no. 5 (2005): 342–59.

Chapter 12: Solo Dining Rx: Share Fare

1. Four elements of the Social Nutrition overeating style are correlated, albeit weakly: 1) eating with family, 2) eating with friends, 3) eating alone, 4) and eating at home at the dining table. When people eat at home and at the dining table it is natural to find that they are also likely to eat with family (r = .42, p <.001), and by themselves less often (r = .62, p <.001).

2. The correlations from our national sample of 5,256 show that those who eat at home at the dining table are less likely to overeat (r = .15, p <.001) and to be overweight (r =.16, p <.001).

3. Deborah Kesten, *The Healing Secrets of Food: A Practical Guide for Nourishing Body, Mind, and Soul* (Novato, CA: New World Library, 2001).

4. Deborah Kesten and Larry Scherwitz, "What's Your Overeating Style? Self-Assessment Quiz," September 15, 2013, http://www.makeweightlosslast.com/2013/05/06/general-introduction/.

5. Deborah Kesten, "The enlightened diet integrative eating e-course." New York: *Spirituality & Health* (December 16, 2002–January 24, 2003).

6. The Social Nutrition element that stood out in terms of decreasing overeating and weight loss was "eating at home at the dining table." The more research participants increased the frequency of eating meals at their dining table, the less they overate (r = .24) and the more weight they lost (r = .30). Eating more frequently with family and friends was also correlated with more weight loss (r = .27; r = .20, respectively), but not as strongly.

7. The Hartman Group, "Table For One: Why We Are Increasingly Eating Alone," May 25, 2016, *Forbes,* https://www.forbes.com/sites/thehartmangroup/2016/05/25/table-for-one-why-we-are-increasingly-eating-alone/#348e53c0616f.

8. Centre for Fathering, "Eat with Your Family Day," accessed February 6, 2019, http://fathers.com.sg/ewyfd/.

9. Hartman Group, *Food and Beverage Analytics: Hartman Eating Occasions Compass,* accessed October 6, 2018, http://store.hartman-group.com/content/food-and-beverage-occasions-compass.pdf.

10. Y. Tani, N. Kondo, et al., "Combined effects of eating alone and living alone on unhealthy dietary behaviors, obesity and underweight in older Japanese adults: results of the JAGES," *Appetite* 95 (December 2015): 1–8.

11. Choi Won-woo and Lee Ki-hun, "People Who Eat Alone More Vulnerable to Obesity," Chosunilbo & Chosun.com, February 15, 2018, http://english.chosun.com/site/data/html_dir/2018/02/15/2018021500536.html.

12. S. Gable S, Y. Chang, J. Krull, et al., "Television Watching and Frequency of Family Meals Are Predictive of Overweight Onset and Persistence in a National Sample of School-Aged Children," *Journal of the Association of Nutrition and Dietetics* 1, no. 107 (January 2007): 53–61.

13. A. Kwon, Y. Yoon, K. Min, et al., "Eating alone and metabolic syndrome: A population-based Korean National Health and Nutrition Examination Survey 2013–2014," Obesity Research & Clinical Practice 12, no. 2 (2018): 146–57.

14. Lim Jeong-Yeo, "Dining alone leads to obesity for Korean millennials," *The Korea Herald/Asia News Network*, November 14, 2018, https://www.thejakartapost.com /life/2018/11/13/dining-alone-leads-to-obesity-for-korean-millennials-study.html.

15. Julie Stewart Wolf and John G. Bruhn, *The Power of Clan: The Influence of Human Relationships on Heart Disease* (New Brunswick, NJ: Transaction, 1993).

16. R. Nerem, J. Murina, J. Levesque, and J. Fredrick Cornhill, "Social Environment as a Factor in Diet-Induced Atherosclerosis," *Science New Series* 208, no. 4451 (1980): 1475–76.

17. Deepak Chopra, *Body, Mind and Soul*, PBS, KQED-TV, San Francisco, March 7, 1995.

18. Larry Scherwitz and Deborah Kesten, "Seven Eating Styles Linked to Overeating, Overweight, and Obesity," *Explore: The Journal of Science and Healing* 1, no. 5 (2005): 342–59.

19. Marion Cunningham, conversation with Deborah Kesten, April 2003.

Chapter 13: In Action: The WPIE Guided Meal Meditation

1. O.M. Aivanhov, *The Yoga of Nutrition* (Frejus, France: Prosveta, 1982).

2. Deepak Chopra, *Ageless Body, Timeless Mind: The Quantum Alternative to Growing Old* (New York: Three Rivers Press, 1993).

3. Jon Kabat-Zinn, *Full Catastrophe Living* (New York: Delacorte Press, 1990), 440.

4. Richard Cavendish, ed., *Man, Myth and Magic: The Illustrated Encyclopedia of Mythology, Religion and the Unknown* (N. Bellmore, NY: Marshall Cavendish Corp., 1987): 12, 1677–1680.

5. Mircea Eliade, ed., *The Encyclopedia of Religion* (New York: Macmillan Publishing Co., 1987), 325.

6. Leo Carver, "10 Powerful Mudras and How to Use Them," The Chopra Center, accessed October 20, 2018, https://chopra.com/articles/10-powerful-mudras-and-how -to-use-them.

Chapter 14: Introduction to the Recipes: Fresh, Whole, Inverse

1. Michael Pollan, *In Defense of Food: An Eater's Manifesto* (New York: Penguin Group, 2008).

2. Larry Scherwitz and Deborah Kesten, "Seven Eating Styles Linked to Overeating, Overweight, and Obesity," *Explore: The Journal of Science and Healing* 1, no. 5 (2005): 342–59.

3. Deborah Kesten and Larry Scherwitz, "Whole Person Integrative Eating: A Program for Treating Overeating, Overweight, and Obesity," *Integrative Medicine: A Clinician's Journal* 14, no. 5 (October/November 2015): 42–50.

4. Deborah Kesten, *The Healing Secrets of Food: A Practical Guide for Nourishing Body, Mind, and Soul* (Novato, CA: New World Library, 2001).

5. K. Tucker, J. Hallfrisch, N. Qiao, et al., "The combination of high fruit and vegetable and low saturated fat intakes is more protective against mortality in aging men than is either

alone: the Baltimore Longitudinal Study of Aging," *J Nutrition* 135, no. 3 (2005): 556–61; F. Hu and W. Willett, "Optimal diets for prevention of coronary heart disease," *Journal of the American Medical Association* 288, no. 20 (November 27, 2002): 2569–2578.

6. K. Steinmetz and J. Potter, "Vegetables, fruit, and cancer prevention: a review," *Journal of American Dietetic Association* 10 (1996): 1027–1039.

7. David Katz, *The Truth About Food: Why Pandas Eat Bamboo, and People Get Bamboozled* (Chesterfield, MO: True Health Initiative, 2018).

8. USDA Economic Research Service, 2009; www.ers.usda.gov/publications/EIB33; www.ers.usda.gov/Data/FoodConsumption/FoodGuideIndex.htm#calories, New York Coalition for Healthy School Food, www.healthyschoolfood.org.

9. Center for Disease Control, "FastStats: Obesity and Overweight," Source: Health, United States, 2013, table 64, accessed July 28, 2014, http://www.cdc.gov/nchs/fastats/obesity-overweight.htm.

10. Ashwani Garg, "Why Diets Fail—The Real 'Magic Weight Loss,'" LinkedIn, June 26, 2014, https://www.linkedin.com/today/post/article/20140626154632-41525622-why-diets-fail-the-real-magic-weight-loss.

11. Y. Progler, "The health impact of a fast food diet: a movie review of "super-size me," *Journal of Research in Medical Sciences* 12 (2007): 275–276.

12. A. Prentice, S. Jebb, "Fast foods, energy density and obesity: a possible mechanistic link," *Obesity Review* 4 (2003): 187–94.

13. S. Stender, J. Dyerberg, and A. Astrup, "High levels of industrially produced trans fat in popular fast foods," *New England Journal of Medicine* 354 (2006): 1650–52.

14. C. Oomen, M. Ocke, E. Feskens, et al., "Association between trans fatty acid intake and 10-year risk of coronary heart disease in the Zutphen Elderly Study: a prospective population-based study," *The Lancet* 357 (2001): 746–751.

15. Cheryl Fryar, "Fast Food Consumption Among Adults in the United States, 2013–2016," NCHS Data Brief No. 322, October 2018, https://www.cdc.gov/nchs/products/databriefs/db322.htm.

16. Centers for Disease Control and Prevention, "Only 1 in 10 Adults Get Enough Fruits or Vegetables," November 16, 2017, https://www.cdc.gov/media/releases/2017/p1116-fruit-vegetable-consumption.html.

17. Roxanne Swentzell and Patricia M. Perea, eds., *The Pueblo Food Experience Cookbook: Whole Food of Our Ancestors*, (New Mexico: Museum of New Mexico Press, 2016).

18. Inez Gomez, "Artist Reclaims Native Culture with Ancestral Foods," *The New Mexican*, accessed August 30, 2018, http://www.santafenewmexican.com/news/community/artist-reclaims-native-culture-with-ancestral-foods/article_21a8e264-1c29-5e25-b0f4-e384a643a2af.html.

19. Deon Ben, "Food as Medicine: The Healing Power of Native foods," Grand Canyon Trust, December 9, 2016, https://www.grandcanyontrust.org/blog/food-medicine-healing-power-native-foods.

20. D. McLaughlin, "The Pueblo Food Experience," Vimeo.com, December 29, 2013.

21. W. Willett, F. Sacks, A. Trichopoulou, G. Drescher, A. Ferro-Luzzi, E. Helsing, et al., "Mediterranean diet pyramid: a cultural model for healthy eating," *American Journal of Clinical Nutrition* 61, no. 6 (1995): 1402-6S.

22. M. Crous-Bou, T. Fung, J. Prescott, et al., "Mediterranean diet and telomere length in Nurses' Health Study: population based cohort study," *British Medical Journal*, no. 20 (2014) 349:6674.

23. S. Olshansky et al., "A Potential Decline in Life Expectancy in the United States in the 21st Century," *New England Journal of Medicine* 352, no. 11 (2005): 1138–45.

24. David Katz, "Sat-Fat Bait and Switch," HuffingtonPost.com, May 5, 2017, https://www .huffingtonpost.com/entry/sat-fat-bait-switch_us_5901f184e4b00acb75f1852as.

25. David Katz, "Dieting in Neverland," LinkedIn.com, August 10, 2018, https://www .linkedin.com/pulse/dieting-neverland-david-l-katz-md-mph-facpm-facp-faclm/.

Epilogue: Our Thoughts on Reshaping the Obesity Crisis in America

1. Deborah Kesten and Larry Scherwitz, "Whole Person Integrative Eating: A Program for Treating Overeating, Overweight, and Obesity," *Integrative Medicine: A Clinician's Journal* 14, no. 5 (October/November 2015): 42–50.

2. Larry Scherwitz and Deborah Kesten, "Seven Eating Styles Linked to Overeating, Overweight, and Obesity," *Explore: The Journal of Science and Healing* 1, no. 5 (2005): 342–59.

3. Deborah Kesten, *The Healing Secrets of Food: A Practical Guide for Nourishing Body, Mind, and Soul* (Novato, CA: New World Library, 2001).

4. Government of Canada, Canada's Food Guide: Canada's Dietary Guidelines, "What are Canada's Dietary Guidelines?" accessed February 12, 2019, https://food-guide.canada .ca/en/guidelines/what-are-canadas-dietary-guidelines/.

5. Laura Calder, "The new Canada Food Guide doesn't just tell us what to eat, but how— and that's a good thing," *The Globe and Mail*, theglobeandmail.com, accessed February 12, 2019, https://www.theglobeandmail.com/opinion/article-the-new-canada-food-guide -doesnt-just-tell-us-what-to-eat-but-how/.

6. Government of Canada, "Eating Well with Canada's Food Guide—A Resource for Educators and Communicators," accessed February 12, 2019, https://www.canada .ca/en/health-canada/services/food-nutrition/reports-publications/eating-well -canada-food-guide-resource-educators-communicators-2007.html.

7. Deborah Kesten and Larry Scherwitz, "White Paper, Whole Person Nutrition: A Re-Visioning of Nutritional Health," May 20, 2013, http://www.makeweightlosslast .com/2013/05/20/whole-person-nutrition-a-re-visioning-of-nutritional-health/.

8. E. Oberg, R. Bradley, J. Allen, and M. McCrory, "Evaluation of a naturopathic nutrition program for type 2 diabetes," *Complementary Therapies in Clinical Practice* 17, no. 3 (2011): 157–161.

9. Ryan Bradley, "Eating habits and diabetes: how we eat may be more important than what we eat," *Diabetes Action* website, June 2011, www.diabetesaction.org/article-eating -habits?rq=ryan%20bradley%202011.

10. Deborah Kesten and Larry Scherwitz, "What's Your Overeating Style? Self-Assessment Quiz," September 15, 2013, http://www.makeweightlosslast.com/2013/05/06 /general-introduction/.

11. Deborah Kesten, Larry Scherwitz, "Holistic, satisfying meals key to optimal nutrition," *Res News Opportunities Sci Theol* 3, no. 3 (November 2002): 11.

12. E. S. Yaseen et al., "Integrative eating style in relation to eating behavior and adiposity in healthy adults," *FASEB Journal* 22, no. 1-supplement (Mar 2008).

13. Deborah Kesten, "Ancient food wisdom meets modern science," *Research News and Opportunities in Science and Theology* 2, no. 7 (2001); Deborah Kesten, Larry Scherwitz, "Holistic, satisfying meals key to optimal nutrition," *Research News and Opportunities in Science and Theology* 3, no. 3 (2002 November): 11.

14. D. Riley, "Integrative Nutrition: Food's Multidimensional Power to Heal," *Explore: The Journal of Science and Healing* 1, no. 5 (2005): 340–41.

15. John Weeks, ed., "Special Focus Issue On Multimodal Approaches In Integrative Health: *Whole Persons, Whole Practices, Whole Systems*," *The Journal of Alternative and Complementary Medicine* 25, no. S1 (March 2019).

Appendix: The Evolution and Science Behind the Overeating Styles

1. Deborah Kesten, *Feeding the Body, Nourishing the Soul: Essentials of Eating for Physical, Emotional, and Spiritual Well-Being* (Berkeley, CA: Conari Press, 1997; Amherst, MA: White River Press, 2007).

2. Deborah Kesten, *The Healing Secrets of Food: A Practical Guide for Nourishing Body, Mind, and Soul* (Novato, CA: New World Library, 2001).

3. Deborah Kesten and Larry Scherwitz, "What's Your Overeating Style? Self-Assessment Quiz," September 15, 2013, https://www.makeweightlosslast.com/2013/05/06/general-introduction/.

4. Deborah Kesten, "The enlightened diet: integrating biological, spiritual, social, and psychological nutrition," *Spirituality & Health* 5 (2003): 29–39.

5. Deborah Kesten, "The enlightened diet integrative eating e-course." New York: *Spirituality & Health* (December 16, 2002–January 24, 2003).

6. Larry Scherwitz and Deborah Kesten, "Seven Eating Styles Linked to Overeating, Overweight, and Obesity," *Explore: The Journal of Science and Healing* 1, no. 5 (2005): 342–59.

7. Max Weber, *Economy and Society* (5th rev. ed.) (Tübingen: Wirtschaft und Gesellschaft, 1972).

8. Thomas Abel, W. Cockerham, G. Lueschen, and G. Kunz (1989), "Health lifestyles and selfdirection in employment among American men: A test of the spillover effect," *Social, Science, and Medicine* 28, 1269–1274.

9. E. Oberg, R. Bradley, J. Allen, and M. McCrory, "Evaluation of a naturopathic nutrition program for type 2 diabetes," *Complementary Therapies and Clinical Practice* 17, no. 3 (2011): 157–61.

10. Ryan Bradley, "Eating habits and diabetes: how we eat may be more important than what we eat," *Diabetes Action* website, June 2011, www.diabetesaction.org/article-eating-habits?rq=ryan%20bradley%202011.

11. E. S. Yaseen, M. M. Gehrke, P. Palmer, I. Kavanaugh, B. Walter, T. Reiss, E. Taylor, and M. McCrory, "Integrative eating style in relation to eating behavior and adiposity in healthy adults," *FASEB Journal* 22, no. 1-supplement (Mar 2008).

12. Deborah Kesten and Larry Scherwitz, "Holistic, satisfying meals key to optimal nutrition," *Research News and Opportunities in Science and Theology* 3, no. 3 (2002): 1.

INDEX

ABOUT THE AUTHORS

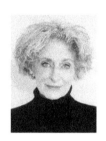 **Deborah Kesten, M.P.H.,** is an international nutrition researcher, award-winning author, and medical and health writer, with a specialty in preventing and reversing obesity and heart disease. A professional health and wellness coach, she was the nutritionist on Dean Ornish, M.D.'s first clinical trial for reversing heart disease through lifestyle changes—the results of which were published in the *Journal of the American Medical Association*—and Director of Nutrition on similar Lifestyle Medicine research at cardiovascular clinics in Europe. She served on the Board of Directors of the American Heart Association, San Francisco, for ten years.

Deborah is Principal Investigator on research about Whole Person Integrative Eating (WPIE), her model and program for treating overeating, overweight, and obesity multidimensionally—physically, emotionally, spiritually, and socially. Her research on WPIE has been published in *Explore: The Journal of Science and Healing* and *Integrative Medicine: A Clinician's Journal*.

Deborah has published more than four hundred nutrition and health articles. Her comprehensive e-course on Whole Person Integrative Eating was featured in *Spirituality & Health* magazine, for which she wrote "The Enlightened Diet" column for two years.

Her first book, *Feeding the Body, Nourishing the Soul*, received the first-place gold award, in the Spirituality category, from the Independent Publisher Book Awards, while an overview of key Whole Person Integrative Eating concepts is the focus of her book *The Healing Secrets of*

288

Food. She is currently a VIP Contributor at Thrive Global. Deborah is married to co-author Larry Scherwitz, Ph.D.

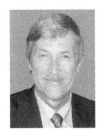 **Larry Scherwitz, Ph.D.,** received his doctorate in Social Psychology from the University of Texas at Austin, trained in psychophysiology at Harvard Medical School, and in behavioral medicine at the University of Wisconsin. He is an international research scientist who has specialized in mind-body research, Lifestyle Medicine, and evidence-based complementary and alternative medicine. His research career includes Director of Research and Co-Principal Investigator with Dean Ornish, M.D., on his heart-disease reversal research, plus research on seven comprehensive Lifestyle Medicine programs with heart patients and their families—four in the United States, three in Europe.

Larry's more recent research includes his groundbreaking discovery linking *self-involvement* to risk of heart attack and death from heart attack, and Co-Principal Investigator on the Whole Person Integrative Eating model and program. Larry has presented his research on self-involvement to His Holiness the Dalai Lama at Mount Sinai Beth Israel Medical Center in New York City. His research has been published in a plethora of prestigious medical journals, from the *Journal of the American Medical Association* and *The Lancet* to *Psychosomatic Medicine.* Larry is married to co-author Deborah Kesten, M.P.H.

CPSIA information can be obtained
at www.ICGtesting.com
Printed in the USA
FSHW020308121019
62910FS

9 781887 043540